Safe Vaccine Administration

Helen Donovan • Helen Bedford
Editors

Safe Vaccine Administration

Practical Guidelines for and by Nurses and Midwives

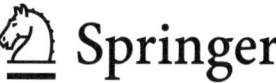

Editors
Helen Donovan
Specialist in immunisation and vaccination
Independent Nurse consultant
London, UK

Helen Bedford
Great Ormond Street Institute of
Child Health
University College London
London, UK

ISBN 978-3-031-92497-2   ISBN 978-3-031-92498-9   (eBook)
https://doi.org/10.1007/978-3-031-92498-9

© Springer Nature Switzerland AG 2025

This work is subject to copyright. All rights are solely and exclusively licensed by the Publisher, whether the whole or part of the material is concerned, specifically the rights of translation, reprinting, reuse of illustrations, recitation, broadcasting, reproduction on microfilms or in any other physical way, and transmission or information storage and retrieval, electronic adaptation, computer software, or by similar or dissimilar methodology now known or hereafter developed.
The use of general descriptive names, registered names, trademarks, service marks, etc. in this publication does not imply, even in the absence of a specific statement, that such names are exempt from the relevant protective laws and regulations and therefore free for general use.
The publisher, the authors and the editors are safe to assume that the advice and information in this book are believed to be true and accurate at the date of publication. Neither the publisher nor the authors or the editors give a warranty, expressed or implied, with respect to the material contained herein or for any errors or omissions that may have been made. The publisher remains neutral with regard to jurisdictional claims in published maps and institutional affiliations.

This Springer imprint is published by the registered company Springer Nature Switzerland AG
The registered company address is: Gewerbestrasse 11, 6330 Cham, Switzerland

If disposing of this product, please recycle the paper.

Foreword

The impact of vaccines in preventing illness, disability and death from once common infectious diseases is unparalleled.

In the UK, provision of vaccination is primarily a nursing role; while the successful roll out of the COVID-19 vaccines involved a wider workforce, nursing staff remained the backbone of delivering this essential service.

This book is written for nurses by nurses and midwives, all with considerable expertise working in different areas of vaccination. It is intended to supplement the existing array of resources available to support best practice in vaccine administration. Although written primarily for a UK nursing audience, many of the issues covered are relevant to nurses in all practice settings and around the world.

As most vaccinators would agree, the actual administration of a vaccine, by injection, orally, or nasally, is only a small part of the overall process. As nurses are widely trusted, they occupy a unique position to provide people with accurate evidence-based information on the benefits and risks of vaccination to support informed decision-making about the vaccines being offered. Nurses can therefore help improve health literacy and vaccine confidence.

Successful vaccine services require an in-depth knowledge of the population or community being served, including cultural awareness, to ensure the service and information offered is tailored appropriately. Vaccinators also need to know which groups in their population may have challenges accessing vaccines and who may have missed them, to plan opportunities to improve access and to enable catch up. To do this effectively requires a highly skilled and motivated nursing workforce.

For many people, vaccination appointments may be the only contact with health services offering a valuable opportunity for wider health assessment as well as for providing health promotion and advice for individuals, families and communities.

Comprehensive, equitable, accessible and affordable vaccination programmes across the life course are key to protecting individuals who are at risk, safeguarding population health and improving the resilience of health systems. Recent political decisions are dramatically changing the global health landscape and raising significant health risks including to vaccination programs and uptake. Global and national health status and security are indivisible and public health funding protects both, which is why we must advocate forcibly for it to be protected.

Wherever you work, vaccination is an exciting, rewarding and ever-expanding area of nursing practice. It is important to understand the development of new vaccine technologies in relation to, for example, cancer as well as the immense benefits to those living with non-communicable diseases. Vaccinations are one of the most powerful interventions we have to improve global health, and delivering on that is quite literally in the hands of nurses right around the world.

Chief Executive Officer International Council of Nurses,   Howard Catton
London, UK

Contents

1 Introduction 1
Helen Donovan
1.1 Value of Vaccines 1
1.2 Vaccine Policy in the UK 3
1.3 UK Vaccination Workforce 4
1.4 Access to Vaccination 4
1.5 Safe Vaccine Service Delivery 5
1.6 Terminology Used in This Book 5
Immunology: Glossary 5
References 6

2 Vaccine Preventable Disease: Introduction 7
Sandra Grieve
2.1 Section 1: Vaccine Preventable Disease in Pregnancy
    and Neonates: Midwives and Vaccination 7
2.2 Section 2: Vaccine Preventable Disease in Infancy and Early
    Childhood 17
2.3 Section 3: Vaccine Preventable Disease in Older Children
    and Young People 25
2.4 Section 4: Vaccine Preventable Disease in Adults 33
2.5 Section 5: Vaccine Preventable Diseases in Travellers
    and Traveller Vaccines 41
2.6 Section 6: Vaccination: Pandemic and Public Health
    Disease Threats 49
References 57

3 Vaccine Development and Onward Management of Vaccine Safety .. 59
Karen Ford and Rachel White
3.1 Introduction 59
3.2 How Do Vaccines Work? 59
3.3 What Is the Ideal Vaccine? 61
3.4 What Are the Different Types of Vaccines? 61
3.5 What Do Vaccines Contain? 62
3.6 Added Ingredients 63

	3.7 How Are Vaccines Tested and Trialled?.	66
	3.8 Phases of Clinical Trials.	68
	3.9 Assessing Immunogenicity of a Vaccine Within Clinical Trials	72
	3.10 Collecting Safety Data Within Clinical Trials	72
	3.11 How Is the Decision to Grant a Licence for a Vaccine Taken?	75
	3.12 Why Is It Important to Know the Possible Expected Adverse Events Following Vaccination?	76
	3.13 How Is the Safety of Vaccines Monitored Once Licensed?.	77
	3.14 How Are Defects in a Vaccine or Batch Reported?.	78
	3.15 How Are Defects in the Devices Used to Administer Vaccines Reported?.	78
	3.16 How Is a Potential Concern over Vaccine Safety Responded to?	79
	References.	81
4	**Being a Safe Practitioner**	83
	Helen Donovan, Sarah Lang, Ashling Kerr, Lindsey Milroy, and Chris Green	
	4.1 Introduction	83
	4.2 Accountability and Delegation.	84
	4.3 Education for Vaccinators	85
	4.4 Varying Learning Needs of Vaccinators.	87
	4.5 Learning and Skills Acquisition.	87
	4.6 Becoming a Vaccinator: Foundation Training	89
	4.7 Continuing Professional Development: Keeping Up-to-Date	90
	4.8 Conclusion	94
	References.	94
5	**Vaccine Storage: "The Cold Chain"**	97
	Laura Craig and Michelle Falconer	
	5.1 Introduction	97
	5.2 Cold Chain Overview.	97
	5.3 Factors Affecting Vaccine Stability	98
	5.4 Impact of Incorrect Storage on Vaccines	98
	5.5 Causes of Vaccine Wastage	100
	5.6 National Recommendations for Vaccine Storage, Distribution and Disposal and Vaccine Incidents.	101
	5.7 Vaccine Incident Scenario	102
	5.8 Conclusion	104
	References.	105
6	**Discussing Vaccination with Parents and Patients**.	107
	Helen Bedford and Helen Donovan	
	6.1 Introduction	107
	6.2 What Is Vaccine Hesitancy?.	107
	6.3 Impact of COVID-19 Pandemic on Public Attitudes to Vaccination.	109
	6.4 The Value of Vaccine Conversations	109

6.5	Timing of Vaccine Information Provision	111
6.6	Frequently Asked Questions	111
6.7	Principles of Discussing Vaccination with Parents and Patients	111
6.8	Conversation Fundamentals	112
6.9	Correcting/Debunking Misinformation	113
6.10	Giving Information About the Diseases and the Vaccines	113
6.11	Unhelpful Strategies	114
6.12	Leaving the Door Open	114
6.13	Conclusion	114
	References	115

7 Principles and Practice of Consent in Relation to Vaccine Administration 117
Helen Donovan, Sarah Lang, David Green, and Chris Green

7.1	Introduction to Consent	117
7.2	Legal Position and Policy	118
7.3	Basic Principles of Consent	118
7.4	Consent Process: Information and Dialogue	119
7.5	Practice Issue: Informed Consent Vs Implied Consent	120
7.6	Informed Consent	120
7.7	Information Resources	122
7.8	Resources in Other Languages	122
7.9	Easy Read Leaflets	122
7.10	Language Interpretation	123
7.11	Literacy Issues	123
7.12	Supporting the Consent Process	123
7.13	Gaining Consent: Practice Based Issues	123
7.14	Can the Individual Provide Consent? Do They Have the Capacity?	123
7.15	Conclusion	127
	References	127

8 Authorisation of Medicines: In Relation to Vaccines 129
David Green, Helen Donovan, Jo Jenkins, and William Malcolm

8.1	Introduction	129
8.2	Legal Administration of Medicines	130
8.3	Classification of Vaccines	130
8.4	Patient Specific Direction (PSD)/Prescription	131
8.5	Alternative Authorisation for Medicines Relevant to Vaccination	132
8.6	Patient Group Directions (PGDs)	133
8.7	Who Can Use a PGD	134
8.8	Written Instructions	135
8.9	National Protocol	136
8.10	Schedule 17 Exemptions for Midwives	136
8.11	Medicines That May Be Administered in Emergency	137
8.12	Conclusion	137
	References	138

9	**Vaccine Administration** 139	

Michelle Falconer, Pauline MacDonald, Laura Craig, Lesley
McFarlane, Debbie Brown, and Jane Dolega-Ossowski

- 9.1 Introduction 139
- 9.2 Before the Vaccine Is Delivered. 140
- 9.3 Understanding the Schedule and Specific Patient Needs. 143
- 9.4 Vaccine Consultation Considerations 144
- 9.5 Medicines Administration: Best Practice Guidance 144
- 9.6 Order in Which Vaccines Are Given 148
- 9.7 Route and Site of Vaccination 148
- 9.8 Injection Site 150
- 9.9 Infants Under the Age of 1 Year. 151
- 9.10 For Children over the Age of 12 Months and Adults. 152
- 9.11 Cautions to Consider Regarding Vaccine Site 154
- 9.12 Giving Multiple Vaccines. 154
- 9.13 Positioning and Reducing Pain 154
- 9.14 Practical Guidelines. Based on "Reducing Pain During Vaccine Injections: Clinical Practice Guideline". 155
- 9.15 Teenagers and Adults. 157
- 9.16 Postvaccination Advice 159
- 9.17 Record-Keeping and Documentation. 160
- References. 160

10 Clinic Management. 163

Pauline MacDonald and Lesley McFarlane

- 10.1 The Importance of Quality Vaccination Clinic Management 163
- 10.2 Knowing the Target Population 164
- 10.3 Best Practice for Clinic Management 165
- 10.4 Prior to the Clinic. 167
- 10.5 During the Clinic 170
- 10.6 Following Vaccination 173
- 10.7 Predeparture. 174
- 10.8 Postvaccination 174
- 10.9 Postvaccination Management 176
- 10.10 Conclusion. 177
- References. 177

11 Infection Prevention and Control Principles for Vaccination. 179

Rose Gallagher

- 11.1 Introduction 179
- 11.2 Maintaining the Quality of the Vaccine 179
- 11.3 Protecting the Healthcare Workers. 179
- 11.4 Best Practice for Prevention of Infection with Vaccine Administration. 181
- 11.5 Summary 185
- References. 185

12	**Maximising Vaccine Uptake: A Population/Community Approach** ... 187
	Louise Letley
	12.1 Introduction 187
	12.2 Health Inequalities 188
	12.3 Know Your Community 188
	12.4 Using Data to Identify Underserved Communities 189
	12.5 Recording Vaccination Data.............................. 189
	12.6 Reducing Inequalities................................... 190
	12.7 Local Knowledge 190
	12.8 Available Evidence...................................... 190
	12.9 Suggestions for Working with Underserved Communities 193
	12.10 Intervention and Evaluation.............................. 195
	12.11 Summary 196
	References... 196

Appendix 1 Resources 199

Appendix 2 Vaccinators: Best Practice/Scope of Practice Considerations..... 203

About the Contributors

Helen Bedford PhD, MSc, BSc, RN, RHV, FiHV, FFPH, FRCPCH, is Professor of Children's Health. Helen joined UCL Institute of Child Health in the late 1980s when MMR vaccine was being introduced to UK. At UCL ICH, the determinants of vaccine uptake and public and health professionals' attitude to vaccines are the main focus of her research. Helen contributes to immunisation training for health care professionals locally and nationally. She is Co-Director of the UCL MSc Paediatrics and Child Health.

Debbie Brown MBE, MSc, BSc (Hons), Dip HE, NMP, RN, is Director of Nursing Primary Care, for South-East London Workforce Development Hub. She has extensive nursing experience in strategic, educational and operational roles primarily in primary care. She is Editor in Chief of *Practice Nursing Journal* and advises at a national level on primary care and nursing standards. She is a Queen's Nurse and was honoured with an MBE for her services to Primary Care Nursing and the NHS.

Laura Craig is a Lead Immunisation Nurse Specialist in the UK Health Security Agency's Immunisation Programmes Division. After gaining clinical experience in a variety of acute paediatric settings and two years carrying out paediatric vaccine trials with the Oxford Vaccine Group, Laura took up her current post in 2002. She is responsible for supporting the implementation of the national immunisation programme through teaching, providing immunisation advice, writing vaccine information and guidance documents and developing national training materials.

Jane Dolega-Ossowski RGN, is a Health Visitor, District Nurse and Practice Nurse for Lewisham Integrated Care System (ICS), leading on vaccination in primary care for practice nurses with a particular interest in training nurses on how to vaccinate and troubleshoot, improving uptake, addressing inequalities and vaccine hesitancy.

Helen Donovan MEd, BSc, RN, RHV, FRSPH, is a Queen's Nurse and has worked in vaccination delivery and policy development as a practice nurse and health visitor and immunisation coordinator in North London. She was the professional lead for public health at the RCN developing guidance and resources for nurses administering vaccines. She now works as an Independent Nurse Consultant in public health, teaching vaccination with a role as Senior Lecturer at the University of Hertfordshire.

Helen Eley RN, is lead immunisation nurse specialist in the UK Health Security Agency, Immunisations programmes division. Initially an infectious diseases nurse, Helen has significant experience in delivering immunisation programmes, as a practice nurse and school aged immunisation nurse, screening and immunisation coordinator and immunisation trainer. In her current role, Helen supports the implementation and maintenance of the national immunisation programmes through training resources, guidance documents and the provision of immunisation advice.

Michelle Falconer MPH, BN (Hons) RN, DN Cert, is a Queens Nurse and an Independent Nurse Consultant in vaccination and immunisation. Michelle has extensive experience in immunisation at a local (Immunisation Coordinator) and nation level, including a specialist improvement role at the Department of Health, Nurse Specialist at UKHSA and recently as a Nurse Consultant at Public Health Scotland. Her experience includes clinical practice, strategy and policy development/implementation, training and education including university post-graduate teaching and vaccine research.

Karen Ford is a Registered Nurse (paediatric nursing) and has a BSc (Hons), MSc degree in Public Health and postgraduate certificate in Medical Education. Karen has worked in clinical vaccine research and immunisation education for the past two decades. She has previously worked in acute paediatrics and neonatal care in the UK, Australia and New Zealand.

Rose Gallagher MBE, is RCN Professional Lead for Sustainability. Rose provides strategic leadership and specialist professional advice to the Royal College of Nursing, its members and key stakeholders across the UK on infection prevention and antimicrobial resistance (AMR) and the implications for nurses and nursing. Her portfolio also includes sustainability, and she leads the College's professional nursing activity on this, in particular the nursing contribution to environmental sustainability. Vaccination is central to the prevention of many preventable infections and benefits communities and healthcare workers alike.

Chris Green is a general and mental health nurse, with experience in acute medicine, ophthalmology, substance-misuse care and school nursing. In 1997, he qualified as a solicitor. He then worked for the RCN for 25 years, representing nurses in professional disciplinary proceedings and inquests, and advising nurses on legal and ethical issues affecting their work.

David Green RN, MPH, PG Cert Health Research, BSc (Hons) Nursing, following a varied nursing career, including general medicine, cardio-thoracic ICU and infection prevention, became an immunisation coordinator in Calderdale in 2008 and has been Nurse Consultant for Immunisations with the national immunisation team at UKHSA since 2014. He is closely involved in the development of PGDs for national vaccination programmes, vaccine incidence management and improving vaccine uptake.

Sandra Grieve RN, RCPS (Glas), is a Travel Health Specialist Nurse with a particular interest in nurse education. She was co-author of guidelines for nurses working in the discipline, emphasising the importance of competence in delivering care to travellers from the UK. With the increasing global spread of infectious diseases and new vaccines becoming available, knowledge of immunisation practice and vaccines related to overseas travel has never been more important.

Greta Hayward RGN, RM, MPH, is a consultant midwife in the Immunisation Programmes Directorate of the UK Health Security Agency. Greta provides expert clinical input to the national public health programmes, aiming to balance the demands of the programmes, against the challenges placed on local services and frontline staff. Greta has worked clinically as a midwife, lectured midwifery students in Borneo and commissioned screening and immunisation services in the East Midlands.

Jo Jenkins is the NHS Specialist Pharmacy Service's Associate Director for Medicines Governance. She leads their Medicines Governance 'Do Once' programme and advises on PGDs and other medicine supply/administration mechanisms for NHS/NHS commissioned services in England. Jo also leads the development of national SPS PGD templates, protocols and governance resources and oversees the publication of resources on PGD/medicines mechanisms development and use on the SPS website.

Ashling Kerr RM, MSc, after registering as a midwife, gained experience working in the Southern Health and Social Care Trust. She has an MSc qualification in Advanced Professional Practice and specialised in Maternal and Child Health. Ashling now works in the Health Protection team in the Public Health Agency, Northern Ireland, providing advice and guidance in response to notifications of infectious disease and leading on the Immunisation and Vaccination workstream.

Sarah Lang RN, MSc, MA, FHEA, MFTM, RCPS (Glas), is a former Immunisation Nurse Specialist. Her primary focus was providing high-quality education and training for immunisers. Her extensive experience of immunisation practice over 20 years provided Sarah with insights into the varied learning needs of immunisers in many contexts. Her areas of practice included primary care, travel clinics and running a vaccine advice services. Sarah currently resides in the USA.

Louise Letley RN, is MSc Nurse Manager (Research) Immunisation and Vaccine Preventable Diseases Division UK Health Security Agency (UKHSA). She is Lead for UKHSA attitudes to vaccination national surveys, joint Lead Investigator on WHO Tailoring Immunisation Programmes (TIP) working with Charedi community in North London. Her special research interests include attitudes to and confidence in vaccination programmes, optimising vaccine uptake, reducing inequalities in uptake and access to vaccination programmes.

Pauline MacDonald ARRC, SRN, BSc (Hons), MSc, FRSPH, is an Independent Consultant Nurse specialising in Immunisation and Infection Prevention, a field she has worked in for over 35 years. For 7 years, Pauline was Nurse Member of the independent advisory committee that advises UK Ministers and the Joint Committee on Vaccination and Immunisation (JCVI). Pauline has experience of immunisation strategy, policy, implementation and delivery from national JCVI level down to local immunisation delivery in primary care, domiciliary and community-based settings.

Briony Mason RM, is Vaccination Manager in NHS England, West Midlands. She qualified as a midwife in 2009 in Manchester and worked in London and Hertfordshire. She set up mass vaccination centres of COVID-19 vaccine in Boston and Lincolnshire and then joined the regional Screening and Immunisation Team, where she led the COVID-19 Vaccination Advice and Response Service for the Midlands. She now manages vaccination coordinators, to deliver immunisation services for routine and selective immunisation services in the West Midlands.

Lesley McFarlane RN, RM, MPH, is Lead Immunisation Nurse Specialist in the Immunisation Programmes Division, UK Health Security Agency. Lesley developed her knowledge of immunisation via posts within practice nursing, health protection and immunisation commissioning and as the Midlands public health nurse lead for the Clinical Advice Response Service for the COVID-19 vaccination programme. She currently works with the national immunisation team, providing advice, writing guidance for healthcare professionals, and developing national training materials and PGDs.

Linzi McIlroy RN, RNT, has an MSc in Health Promotion and Public Health, and BSC (Hons) and Advanced Diploma in Teaching Studies for Nurses. Currently she is Senior Nurse Professional Practice in RCN Northern Ireland. She is the lead for primary care nursing and facilitates education programmes for nurses working in Primary Care.

Lindsey Milroy RGN, BSc (HONS), MSc, Principal Educator NHS Education for Scotland, Edinburgh, Registered Nurse with acute care experience, following a period of time in quality improvement moved into the sphere of post graduate education. Currently leads vaccination workforce education development, in collaboration with the Scottish Vaccination and Immunisation Programme.

Clare Powell BSc Hons, SCPHN (HV), RSCN, RN, is Specialist Immunisation Nurse, training Lead Vaccine Preventable Disease programme, Public health, Wales.

Rachel White RN, graduated with a Diploma in Paediatric Nursing in 2007 and has worked as an RN in many paediatric settings, including high dependency and intensive care. Rachel has spent the last 10 years in clinical research in many trials surrounding new and improved vaccines.

Introduction

Helen Donovan

In the UK, the majority of vaccine services are delivered by nursing and midwifery staff, in contrast with many other countries where vaccination is often a medical procedure. This book is written by and intended primarily for nurses, midwives and others involved in the delivery of vaccination programmes to share best vaccination practice.

The book covers vaccination practice across all areas of nursing and midwifery including school nursing and health visiting. It will support the delivery of a safe clinic environment that is accessible to all sectors of the population—alongside the importance of having a skilled and knowledgeable workforce to ensure safe and effective practice and managing questions from parents and the public.

It is intended as an adjunct to, not a replacement for, other resources to which we include references with links to trusted and useful websites to support signposting.

1.1 Value of Vaccines

Vaccination is widely recognised as a highly effective public health intervention, ranking second only to the provision of clean water in its impact on disease prevention. The use of vaccines to protect individuals from infectious diseases and reduce the risk of serious complications and death has had a significant impact on our health. It is estimated that 3.5–5 million deaths a year are averted as the result of vaccination (WHO World Health Organization 2024). Despite its success, vaccines do not reach everyone; it is estimated that over 12 million children remain completely unvaccinated (zero-dose children) (GAVI 2024). The reasons for this are

---

General support and contribution from: Linzi McIlroy – RCN Northern Ireland; Clare Powell – Public Health Wales

---

H. Donovan (✉)
Specialist in Immunisation and Vaccination, Independent Nurse Consultant, London, UK

© Springer Nature Switzerland AG 2025
H. Donovan, H. Bedford (eds.), *Safe Vaccine Administration*,
https://doi.org/10.1007/978-3-031-92498-9_1

complex but improving access to vaccination remains a WHO priority. The WHO Immunization Agenda 2030 sets out a vision for vaccination with a global strategy to leave no one behind (WHO 2020).

The majority of routine vaccines are recommended for and given to children to provide protection as early in life as possible. However, it is increasingly important to consider vaccination for people throughout their lives. Chapter 2 discusses the rationale for giving vaccines to people at different ages and stages in their lives.

It is beyond the scope of this book to go into detail on how vaccines work—this is covered in the Green Book Chap. 1. It is important to note, however, that the various vaccines work in different ways, and this is often an important consideration for the overall aim of the specific vaccine programme—whether this is to eradicate a disease, control it, or minimise the impact to those most at risk.

Vaccines work by protecting the individual, by stimulating an immune response, so the individual can fight the infection more effectively—this is discussed further in Chap. 3. This may not necessarily prevent all infection but may prevent them getting more severe disease.

Vaccines arguably have an even greater value in protecting the wider population. Herd or community immunity occurs in a population, where you have significant numbers who are vaccinated and as such a reduced number who are susceptible to a disease, meaning it is less likely for those who are not protected come into contact with the disease.

Some vaccines have the added value of stopping the transmission and spread of infection. Many infections are spread between individuals who carry the organism themselves but have no or very mild symptoms. For example, the meningococcal and pneumococcal conjugate vaccines also reduce the carriage of the organisms for which they are designed. This means therefore that even those not vaccinated have benefitted, with reduction in carriage the organism is less likely transmitted.

Vaccination in the UK. In the UK, a comprehensive vaccine schedule is offered to people throughout their life course from pregnancy to older age. The schedule is increasingly complex and changes regularly in response to changes in disease epidemiology as a result of vaccination, with different dosing schedules, changes to vaccine supply, or, as new vaccines become available, programmes to introduce them to the schedule are developed. Chapter 3 discusses the elements involved in developing vaccine programmes including vaccine trials.

Generally, the uptake of vaccines across the UK population is relatively high, and the incidence of many once common infectious diseases has become vanishingly rare. Uptake has, however, been declining over the last 10 years, and significant challenges remain for vaccine programmes to attain and sustain high uptake. The very success of vaccination programmes in reducing disease means that maintaining high vaccine uptake can become challenging. In the context of low or no disease, effectively addressing public perceptions about the necessity of vaccination to protect against diseases, they don't recognise relative to perceived concerns over the safety of vaccines. Chapter 6 discusses the importance of vaccine conversations.

During and since the COVID pandemic, vaccine acceptance has declined in many countries. This decline, following a period of extremely low incidence of other infections due to the public health measures introduced in the pandemic to limit infection spread, has left many children susceptible, resulting in outbreaks of measles and pertussis in the UK and other countries—in addition to sustaining the established vaccination programmes and supporting the expansion of the routine programme, for example, with vaccines for respiratory syncytial virus (RSV) and varicella (chickenpox). Vaccines are also essential to tackle the challenge of emerging infections such as Ebola, MPOX, or coronaviruses.

1.2 Vaccine Policy in the UK

1.2.1 Joint Committee in Vaccination (JCVI) and UK Governments

In the UK, the Joint Committee on Vaccination and Immunisation (JCVI), an expert advisory committee, advises the UK government on vaccination. The remit is:

"To advise UK health departments on immunisations for the prevention of infections and/or disease following due consideration of the evidence on the burden of disease, on vaccine safety and efficacy and on the impact and cost effectiveness of immunisation strategies. To consider and identify factors for the successful and effective implementation of immunisation strategies. To identify important knowledge gaps relating to immunisations or immunisation programmes where further research and/or surveillance should be considered". (JCVI 2013 p4 point 6)

The JCVI has no statutory responsibility to provide advice to Ministers in Scotland or Northern Ireland; however, health departments from these countries may choose to accept the Committee's advice or recommendations.

JCVI provides advice and recommendations for the national vaccination programmes. This is based on scrutiny of available evidence and literature, both published and unpublished; analysis of epidemiological data of disease incidence; consideration of the economic and health benefits of specific vaccinations; and the benefit of making changes to the schedule. The UK government makes decisions about policy and ensures this is implemented. The recommended schedule is broadly the same across all UK countries (JCVI 2023).

1.2.2 Immunisation Against Infectious Disease: The "Green Book"

This document sets out the detailed policy and procedures for vaccination and the vaccine schedule for each infectious disease.

The "Green Book" is available as individual chapters via the Immunisation section of the GOV. UK website (UKHSA (On Line) n.d.).

Part I of the Green Book (Chaps. 1–12) addresses the principles, practice and procedures for vaccination.

Part II covers the diseases and vaccinations with each detailed in a separate chapter. The chapters are updated regularly to reflect changes to individual vaccine programmes or amendments to vaccine procedures and new chapters added to reflect new vaccine programmes.

Throughout this book, the relevant chapters of the "Green Book" will be referenced as UK Health Security Agency (UKHSA) online, Immunisation Against Infectious Disease, and they should be accessed on line via the GOV.UK website: immunisation-against-infectious-disease-the-green-book.

1.2.3 The Medicines and Healthcare Products Regulatory Agency (MHRA)

The MHRA is an executive agency of the Department of Health and Social Care (DHSC), Medicines and Healthcare products Regulatory Agency - GOV.UK, responsible for the regulation and the legislation for medicines applies across all UK countries. Chapter 8 describes in more detail the medicines legislation in relation to vaccination.

1.3 UK Vaccination Workforce

In the UK, vaccination remains a core function for general practice, community and school aged immunisation services (SAIS). Yet, its routine nature can mean that it is sometimes viewed as "just giving an injection" with the skills and knowledge needed to deliver a safe and effective service not given appropriate priority.

The increasing complexity of the schedule with the addition of new vaccines and schedule alterations makes it essential for vaccinators to keep up to date. The importance of continual practice development and the training requirements for vaccinators is discussed in Chap. 4.

1.4 Access to Vaccination

The contracts for providing vaccination and how services are configured differ across the UK. It is beyond the scope of this book to go into the detail of how individual services are designed. It is, however, essential for the key elements to be in place to ensure all those eligible for the recommended vaccines are able to access them. This is addressed in Chap. 12.

The UK policy reflects the WHO assertion that vaccination is an indisputable human right (WHO World Health Organization 2024) and individuals have the right to those vaccines recommended under the NHS (NHS 2023). Vaccination in the UK is an individual choice people need to consent to receive. The principles of consent are discussed in Chap. 7.

1.5 Safe Vaccine Service Delivery

Vaccine services are managed differently across the UK dependent on local needs and the governance and management systems. However, there are some core principles and standards required to ensure vaccine services are safe and effective. Vaccines must be stored according to the manufacturer's licence; these requirements are discussed in Chap. 5. Vaccine administration is discussed in Chap. 9, clinic management in Chap. 10 and safe infection prevention and control in relation to vaccine services in Chap. 11. The UKHSA Quality criteria for an effective Immunisation programme, provides a useful guide for the key elements required for the implementation and delivery of a safe, equitable, high quality, effective and efficient immunisation services able to respond to the needs of vaccine recipients and wider population (UKHSA 2025).

1.6 Terminology Used in This Book

Parent/carer includes guardians or anyone accompanying someone for vaccination.

Nursing staff includes all nurses and midwives as well as nursing support staff involved in vaccination.

Acknowledgements With thanks to all the authors and contributors to the book chapters for their time and expertise in putting the resource together

The photographs used in the book have been organised by colleagues in Southeast London: Debbie Brown, primary care nurse consultant for Lewisham CCG, and Jane Dolega-Ossowski, practice nurse advisor for Lewisham ICS. The patients or parents (mothers) have given permission for the photographs to be used for the purpose of this health related book. We give thanks to the patients and staff for their consent.

Immunology: Glossary[1]

The innate system An in-built protection from barriers such as the skin, acidity in the gut, tears, etc. The body's first line of defence.

The adaptive system Whereby the body develops specific protection through a complex arrangement between specialised blood cells and chemical mediators to develop immunity specific to a particular substance.

Immunisation The process whereby an individual is protected from a specific antigen—this can include any germ which causes disease, bacteria or virus. It can be achieved through natural infection or receipt of a vaccine.

---

[1] It is beyond the scope of this book to cover the process of immunology in detail, but an understanding of the process and what this means in relation to vaccination is essential. The following provides definitions of the relevant terminology and some key resources for further reading:

The immune system is complex but essentially consists of the following:

Antigen: A toxin or other foreign substance which induces an immune response in the body, especially the production of antibodies.

Vaccination The process of giving a vaccine which produces specific antibodies for the particular disease/infection and provides immunity.

Antibody: Also called immunoglobulins, found in the blood or other body fluids. They are produced in response to an antigen either from infection with a disease or from a vaccine.

Immunity Acquired after an individual has had a disease or after vaccination. The individual makes antibodies which are memorised by the cells so it can produce specific antibodies for this infection quickly if the individual is exposed to the antigen again.

Vaccine Monovalent—including one antigen
Multivalent—including two or more antigens

References

GAVI. Reaching zero dose children. https://www.gavi.org/our-alliance/strategy/phase-5-2021-2025/equity-goal/zero-dose-children-missed-communities (accessed 04/11/2024)

JCVI (2023) Code of Practice (Accessed 04/11/2024) https://www.gov.uk/government/uploads/system/uploads/attachment_data/file/224864/JCVI_Code_of_Practice_revision_2013_-_final.pdf

NHS (2023) NHS Constitution for England https://www.gov.uk/government/publications/the-nhs-constitution-for-england [Accessed 04/11/24]

UKHSA (On Line): (n.d.) The Green Book Immunisation against infectious disease https://www.gov.uk/government/collections/immunisation-against-infectious-disease-the-green-book [04/11/24]

UKHSA (2025) Guidance: Quality criteria for an effective immunisation programme https://www.gov.uk/government/publications/quality-criteria-for-an-effective-immunisation-programme (07/07/2025)

WHO World Health Organization (2024). Vaccines and Immunization. https://www.who.int/health-topics/vaccines-and-immunization#tab=tab_1 (accessed 04/11/24)

WHO (2020) Immunization Agenda 2030: A Global Strategy To Leave No One Behind https://www.who.int/publications/m/item/immunization-agenda-2030-a-global-strategy-to-leave-no-one-behind (accessed 31/10/2024)

Vaccine Preventable Disease: Introduction

2

Sandra Grieve

2.1 Section 1: Vaccine Preventable Disease in Pregnancy and Neonates: Midwives and Vaccination

Helen Donovan[1], Greta Hayward[2], Briony Mason[3]
 [1] London, UK
 [2] Design, Implementation and Clinical Guidance Division, UK Health Security Agency, London, UK
 [3] NHS England, West Midlands, Birmingham, UK

> **Abstract**
> This section considers the role of midwives and the changing use of vaccines in pregnancy to protect neonates and pregnant women.
> Infectious diseases in pregnancy or in the immediate postnatal period can be associated with an increased risk of death and long-term complications for both the mother and her unborn baby/the newborn infant.
> Vaccine programmes offered in pregnancy or to infants in the neonatal period include the following:
>
> - Pregnancy programmes to protect against influenza, COVID-19, pertussis (whooping cough) and respiratory syncytial virus (RSV).
> - Programmes designed specifically to protect very young infants at increased risk of infection: BCG vaccine for protection against tuberculosis and hepatitis B vaccine.
>
> (continued)

S. Grieve (✉)
London, UK

- Pregnancy and preconception discussions also provide a wider opportunity to make sure women are up to date with all the vaccines recommended in the routine programme. All women should be protected against rubella, before pregnancy, with two doses of the measles, mumps and rubella (MMR) vaccine. Women who have not had MMR vaccine should be offered the vaccine postnatally to protect future pregnancies.

Keywords: vaccination in pregnancy, infectious disease in pregnancy

2.1.1 Introduction

Vaccination is an important intervention to protect pregnant women from some infections which put the mother, the fetus and/or neonate at increased risk of more severe outcomes. It also provides protection to the newborn infant at a time when they are most vulnerable to severe outcomes. Pregnancy will often be the first time many people will become aware of the routine immunisation schedule and presents a valuable opportunity to discuss the importance of vaccination not only to protect the pregnant woman but also her child in its early weeks of life.

Midwives have always been involved in providing advice on immunisation and participating in early discussions with parents about the vaccines recommended for them and their babies. Using opportunities during pregnancy to provide women and their partners with the information and support they need to make decisions for the future health of their baby is important. Vaccination in pregnancy is now a routine part of antenatal care, with women being offered vaccines during their planned appointments, and it represents the start of the vaccination life course, for the infant but also to protect the pregnant woman.

2.1.2 Maternal Acquired Immunity

Maternally derived passive immunity develops in unborn babies during the pregnancy. The mother's antibodies, acquired either from a past infection or vaccination, are transferred to the unborn child through the placenta (Amirthalingam et al 2022). These antibodies provide the newborn infant with passive immunity against some bacterial and viral infections from birth. Although immunity is short-lived, it will generally provide the infant with some protection until they can commence their own vaccine course at 8 weeks of age. Some passively acquired antibodies, such as those that protect against measles, last for longer.

The recognition that infants are protected from subsequent infection through their mother's immunity is not new:

- Investigations into the 1846 measles outbreak on the Faro Islands demonstrated that the immunity they gained from their mothers protected infants against measles (Moss 2018).

The use of vaccines given to pregnant women to achieve passive immunity is also well established.

- Protection of babies through the immunity acquired from vaccination of mothers during pregnancy goes back to 1879 where the infants of mothers given the smallpox vaccine were shown to be protected (De Martino 2016).
- Neonatal tetanus continues to be a significant problem in certain parts of the world. In 1989, the World Health Organization (WHO) established the Maternal and Neonatal Tetanus Elimination (MNTE) programme, to provide routine tetanus toxoid vaccination for pregnant women alongside the promotion of clean deliveries and cord care. The WHO estimated that in 2021 there had been an 88% reduction in deaths in newborns from neonatal tetanus compared with 2000 (WHO 2024), but this still represented 24,000 newborn deaths.

2.1.3 Infection in Pregnancy and Vaccination

Pregnancy causes changes to the normal immune response which may result in an altered susceptibility for the women and fetus and an increased risk of serious outcomes from certain infections (Jamieson et al 2006) such as influenza and COVID-19. It is recognised that many women have anxieties about vaccination in pregnancy and will have questions about their necessity and safety for themselves as well as their baby (Campbell et al 2015); similarly women have reported concerns accepting the COVID-19 vaccines (Skirrow et al 2021).

As generally the advice in pregnancy is to be cautious about taking medication in case it affects the developing fetus, it is understandable that pregnant women will have questions and concerns about vaccination. It is thus essential for women to be provided with clear, consistent advice and information on vaccine safety and the rationale for vaccination. Midwives are pivotal in giving this information and supporting women in their vaccination decisions. However, midwives may have their own concerns about vaccination in pregnancy and require education and training to improve their knowledge and confidence (Vishram 2017).

Pregnant women will ordinarily be excluded from vaccine trials, and so most vaccines will not have been actively tested on pregnant women, due to any potential risk to the pregnancy and/or unborn infant. When a vaccine comes into routine use, the manufacturers' summary of product characteristics (SmPC) usually advises using with caution in pregnancy. The rationale for this advice is because of a *lack* of safety information rather than any proven risk associated with vaccination in pregnancy; this can be a cause of anxiety to women and midwives. However, because pregnant women are sometimes inadvertently vaccinated (often before they know they are pregnant) or where vaccines have been given after careful consideration of the risks, there is a body of evidence. This has been reviewed and evaluated by the WHO Global Advisory Committee for Vaccine Safety (GACVS) (WHO 2014). The review found no evidence of adverse pregnancy outcomes from vaccination with inactivated vaccines, and therefore, where it is appropriate, vaccination should be available in pregnancy. The report also concluded that although live vaccines pose a theoretical risk to the fetus, there is a substantial body of literature describing their safety.

Vaccination is also important to ensure women are protected against specific infections before they become pregnant. For example, rubella infection in the first 16 weeks of pregnancy is associated with a high risk of major congenital abnormalities (congenital rubella syndrome). Midwives should check **MMR status of all pregnant women** and refer unvaccinated and partially vaccinated women to their GP practice to catch up after they deliver.

The benefits of vaccination are always assessed in relation to the specific threat caused by the disease in comparison with perceived risks and the feasibility of ensuring the vaccine is available to all pregnant women.

2.1.4 Specific Vaccines and Screening Recommended in the UK During Pregnancy

The following vaccines, or screening for vaccination, are recommended routinely in the UK for pregnant women or newborn infants.

As for all UK vaccine programmes, the details are available in the "Green Book" and specific programme guidance in guidance for health care professionals

2.1.4.1 Influenza Vaccination

Influenza is more likely to cause severe illness in pregnant women than those who are not pregnant. The reason for this is thought to be due to the normal physiological changes that occur during pregnancy, altered heart rate, oxygen consumption and immune response. The inactivated influenza vaccine is offered to pregnant women during the flu season (September to March) to protect the women themselves and provide passive immunity to their baby in the first few months of life. The changing nature of influenza viruses means that the vaccines are modified according to the latest virus strains and in line with World Health Organisation (WHO) recommendations. Immunisation must be repeated with every pregnancy (UKHSA annual flu programme—online).

The vaccine can be given at any stage of pregnancy and helps protect against influenza and its complications, including maternal pneumonia, premature birth, low birth weight and in rare cases maternal mortality. Influenza can also be serious for neonates, and passive immunity acquired from a vaccinated mother also provides some immunity for the infant (WHO 2014; and UKHSA 2023).

2.1.4.2 Pertussis Vaccination

Pertussis or whooping cough disease can be fatal, particularly in babies who are too young to be protected by the primary immunisation schedule. In 2011–2012, there was a marked increase in the number of cases of pertussis reported in England—a similar rise in cases was also seen in many other countries. This rise saw the tragic death of a small number of infants (UKHSA 2021).

In 2012, an emergency programme of maternal pertussis immunisation was introduced to help prevent infant deaths. Maternal vaccination boosts the existing maternal antibodies which cross the placenta and provide passive immunity protection to the baby for the first few months, until they can receive pertussis vaccine as part of the routine childhood schedule. The maternal pertussis vaccine programme was made permanent following advice from the Joint Committee of Vaccination and Immunisation in 2019 (UKHSA 2021).

The vaccine is offered to all pregnant women in each pregnancy. Women should be offered the vaccine between weeks 16 and 32 of pregnancy, usually around the time of the fetal anomaly scan (20 weeks). Women may still be immunised after week 32 of pregnancy until delivery. This may not, however, offer a high enough level of passive protection to the baby, particularly if they are born preterm (UKHSA 2024a). Women who miss the vaccine while they are pregnant can still have it up to 8 weeks after birth when their baby is old enough to receive their first pertussis containing vaccine, to help minimise risk of infection from the mother to baby.

The data show the maternal vaccine programme, introduced in October 2012, has reduced the number of pertussis infections. Sadly, however, we still see deaths in babies from pertussis—most of these are in infants whose mothers did not receive the pertussis vaccine or were vaccinated late in their pregnancy. In 2024, we have seen a significant increase in cases of pertussis in all age groups including babies who often have worse outcomes (UKHSA 2024b). It is imperative women are advised and encouraged to have the vaccine early enough in their pregnancy to afford maximum protection. There are now data from over a million pregnancies of the safety of maternal pertussis vaccination into childhood (Laverty et al 2021).

2.1.4.3 Checking MMR Vaccine Status

The combined measles, mumps and rubella (MMR) vaccine was introduced into the UK in 1988 with a second dose added to the schedule in 1996. A single rubella vaccine for girls only was introduced in 1973. Rubella is normally a mild illness but can be very serious if caught in pregnancy, particularly in the early stages when it can cause serious complications for the fetus as a result of the congenital rubella syndrome (CRS) or lead to miscarriage. The vaccine is very effective, providing protection in 95–100% of vaccinees (UKHSA Green Book, "Rubella" chapter). Since the introduction of universal MMR vaccination, infections from rubella in the UK are now very rare. Those most at risk are likely to be non-born-UK women who have not had MMR vaccine and come from rubella endemic countries (Bukasa et al 2018). Women should be asked about their MMR vaccination history during preconception opportunities such as cervical screening or family planning consultations. They should also be asked during the antenatal period to check they have had the recommended two doses of vaccine.

If a pregnant woman has not had the recommended two doses of MMR vaccine, as live vaccines are not recommended in pregnancy, she should be offered the missing doses postpartum at the postnatal check when her baby starts the vaccination course. This is to provide protection against rubella in future pregnancies.

2.1.4.4 Hepatitis B Screening and Vaccination

The World Health Organization (WHO) has classified hepatitis as an international public health challenge. Hepatitis B is an infection of the liver which can have very serious consequences; around 20–25% of those with chronic infection will develop progressive liver disease and potentially cirrhosis of the liver (UKHSA Green Book, "Hepatitis B" chapter). Although rates of infection across the UK population are relatively low, certain groups are at particular high risk of infection and ongoing disease. Infants born to mothers who have screened positive for hepatitis B virus (HBV) in pregnancy, or whose mothers have acute hepatitis B infection during their pregnancy, are at high risk of acquiring infection at or around the time of delivery (vertical transmission)—these infants have a 90% risk of developing chronic infection (UKHSA 2023).

The Infectious Diseases in Pregnancy Screening (IDPS) hepatitis B pathway includes a robust process to ensure the following:

- Timely antenatal screening for the presence of hepatitis B infection. Antenatal screening is offered to all pregnant women with appropriate counselling. The screening includes assessing for the presence of hepatitis B surface antigen (HBsAg) to indicate infection.
- Women identified as having hepatitis B infection should be referred for ongoing appropriate clinical care and during pregnancy and at delivery.
- Optimal safe delivery of the infant.
- Infants identified at being at risk of vertical transmission of hepatitis B virus infection are given a selective accelerated hepatitis B vaccination programme in addition to the hepatitis B vaccine provided as part of the routine childhood schedule.
- Subsequent screening of the infants at 1 year of age, with dry blood spot (DBS) sampling for HBsAg, to ensure they have not acquired hepatitis B infection.
- Onward prompt referral of any infants identified as having HBsAg, hepatitis B infection.

The guidance also recommends a further safeguard where the infant is at risk of exposure to the virus from another member of the household who is known to be infected. In these situations, a monovalent dose of hepatitis B vaccine can be offered before discharge from hospital to provide some protection before the child's routine immunisations begin (UKHSA 2023).

This comprehensive pathway crosses maternity, primary care and specialist services. Midwives play a vital role in the delivery of the pathway and in counselling parents on its importance. As a result of this robust screening and vaccination programme, the UK has achieved the WHO target of demonstrating the elimination of mother to child transmission (MTCT) with 0.1% of infants testing positive on DBS for HBsAg.

2.1.5 Neonatal BCG

The neonatal BCG vaccination programme is aimed at protecting babies and young children most at risk of exposure to tuberculosis. The Bacillus Calmette-Guérin (BCG) vaccine, when given to infants, will help minimise the risk of disseminated TB, meningitis and septicaemia.

The selective immunisation programme is to offer BCG vaccine, by 28 days of age:

- To all infants with a parent or grandparent born in a country where the yearly incidence of TB is 40 per 100,000 or greater
- To all infants living in areas of the UK where the yearly incidence of TB is 40 per 100,000 or greater

Severe combined immunodeficiency (SCID) screening was introduced as an evaluative roll-out programme in 2021 (UKHSA 2021). In parts of England, SCID screening has been added to the newborn bloodspot screening (NBS) programme for babies at day 5. As BCG is a live vaccine and contraindicated in those who are immunosuppressed, it shouldn't be offered to babies known to have SCID. The BCG vaccine programme requires babies' SCID results are checked prior to giving the BCG vaccine at around 28 days (UKHSA 2021a).

Models of BCG vaccination delivery differ across the country, but midwives have a vital role in identifying eligible babies and recommending vaccination where appropriate.

2.1.6 COVID-19 Vaccine

Pregnancy does not specifically increase the chance of contracting SARS-CoV2 infection. However, if caught, particularly in the third trimester, there is an increased risk of severe illness requiring intensive care or advanced respiratory support. This greatly increases the chance of premature birth and the associated complications for women and their babies (Knight et al 2020). As with most vaccines, those for COVID-19 were not initially tested on pregnant women. However, since their introduction in 2020, millions of pregnant women have received COVID-19 vaccines globally. There is very good evidence for their safety and the protection they provide against severe disease for pregnant women and their babies (UKHSA 2021).

Pregnant women should be encouraged to accept the COVID-19 vaccines when eligible and as recommended (UKHSA Green Book, "COVID-19" chapter).

Midwives have a crucial role in providing clear advice to women and their families that vaccines for COVID-19 are safe and effective in protecting themselves and their baby from severe disease and hospitalisation. They also have a crucial role to play in ensuring pregnant women can access all recommended vaccines (RCOG 2022).

2.1.7 Respiratory Syncytial Virus (RSV)

Over the last few years, there have been vaccine options developed for respiratory syncytial virus (RSV), a common virus which causes cold like symptoms. Most children will be infected by RSV by the time they are 2 years of age, and individuals frequently get reinfections as they get older. The main burden of infection from RSV is in infants with bronchiolitis and respiratory complications. Before the RSV vaccine programme commenced, the virus was estimated to cause over 30,000 hospitalisations in children under 5 years of age and 20–30 deaths in children, every year (Green Book, "RSV" chapter).

A monoclonal antibody preparation to protect against RSV is recommended for high-risk infants to provide immediate passive immunity.

An RSV vaccine programme to reduce the incidence and severity of RSV disease in infants has been introduced from September 2024 following JCVI recommendation (JCVI 2023). The RSV vaccine should be offered to all pregnant women from 28 weeks' gestation in each pregnancy. While most women will have been exposed to RSV infection during their lives, antibody levels acquired from natural infection will not provide sufficient protection to their infant. Giving an RSV vaccine from week 28 of every pregnancy will temporarily boost the mother's antibody levels so that a high level of RSV antibodies can be transferred across the placenta providing passive protection to the infant against RSV for the first months of life, even where babies are born prematurely (UKHSA 2024a). There is a separate programme to vaccinate those over 75 years of age and reduce the burden of RSV to older people (see the section on vaccines in adults in this chapter).

2.1.8 Conclusion

Pregnancy has always been recognised as an ideal time to provide advice and support to promote healthy lifestyle and behaviours for the whole family to give children the best start in life (PHE 2016). Vaccination in pregnancy against specific infections is proven safe and highly effective, and midwives are ideally placed to discuss and promote vaccination throughout pregnancy and during the immediate postnatal period. They need to ensure they know where to access the most recent information on new vaccines including the rationale for their inclusion, in the online version of the Green Book *Immunisation Against Infectious Diseases* (UKHSA Green Book online).

The offer of vaccination in pregnancy is likely to expand. Further to the latest addition of RSV vaccination of pregnant women for infant protection, there are other potential vaccines in development such as group B streptococcus (Oxford vaccine knowledge project Group B Streptococcus online).

References

Amirthalingam H, Campbell H, Ribeiro S, Stowe J, Tessier E, Litt D, Fry NK, Andrews N. (2022) Optimization of Timing of Maternal Pertussis Immunization From 6 Years of Postimplementation Surveillance Data in England. *Clinical Infectious Diseases*, 76 (3), pp1129–e1139 https://doi.org/10.1093/cid/ciac651 [Accessed August 2024]

Bukasa, A., Campbell, H., Brown, K., Bedford, H., Ramsay, M., Amirthalingam, G. and Tookey, P., 2018. Rubella infection in pregnancy and congenital rubella in United Kingdom, 2003 to 2016. *Eurosurveillance*, 23(19), pp.17-00381.

Campbell et al (2015): Attitudes to immunisation in pregnancy among women in the UK targeted by such programmes https://www.magonlinelibrary.com/doi/full/10.12968/bjom.2015.23.8.566 [Accessed March 2023]

De Martino M (2016): Dismantling the Taboo against Vaccines in Pregnancy International Journal of Molecular Sciences 17(6): 894. Dismantling the Taboo against Vaccines in Pregnancy - PMC (nih.gov) (accessed March 20230

Knight, M. et al. (2020): Obstetric Surveillance System SARS-CoV-2 Infection in Pregnancy Collaborative Group. 2020. Characteristics and outcomes of pregnant women admitted to hospital with confirmed SARS-CoV-2 infection in UK: national population based cohort study. British Medical Journal BMJ. 369: https://doi.org/10.1136/bmj.m2107.

Jamieson DJ, Theiler RN, Rasmussen SA. (2006): Emerging infections and pregnancy. Emerging *Infectious Diseases Journal*, 12(11):1638–1643.

JCVI (2023) Independent report Respiratory syncytial virus (RSV) immunisation programme for infants and older adults: JCVI full statement, 11 September 2023 https://www.gov.uk/government/publications/rsv-immunisation-programme-jcvi-advice-7-june-2023/respiratory-syncytial-virus-rsv-immunisation-programme-for-infants-and-older-adults-jcvi-full-statement-11-september-2023

Laverty et al (2021): Health Outcomes in Young Children Following Pertussis Vaccination During Pregnancy. Pediatrics. 147(5): https://pubmed.ncbi.nlm.nih.gov/33875535/

Moss W, (2018): Measles in Vaccinated Individuals and the Future of Measles Elimination. *Clinical Infectious Diseases*, V 67(9): Pages 1320–1321.

Oxford Vaccine Knowledge Group. Group B streptococcus (on line) https://www.ovg.ox.ac.uk/research/group-b-streptococcus [Accessed March 2023]

Royal College of Obstetricians and Gynaecologists (RCOG) (2022): COVID-19 vaccines, pregnancy, and breastfeeding FAQs. Available at: COVID-19 vaccines, pregnancy and breastfeeding FAQs | RCOG. Accessed March 2023.

Skirrow H, Barnett S, Bell S, Riaposova L, Mounier-Jack S, Kampmann B and Holder B (2021): Women's views on accepting COVID-19 vaccination during and after pregnancy, and for their babies: A multi-methods study in the UK BMC Pregnancy and Childbirth https://www.medrxiv.org/content/10.1101/2021.04.30.21256240v1.full [Accessed March 2023]

PHE (2019) Laboratory confirmed cases of pertussis in England: annual report for 2019 https://assets.publishing.service.gov.uk/government/uploads/system/uploads/attachment_data/file/881380/hpr0820_PRTSSS_annual.pdf [Accessed March 2023]

PHE (2016): Health matters: giving every child the best start in life https://www.gov.uk/government/publications/health-matters-giving-every-child-the-best-start-in-life/health-matters-giving-every-child-the-best-start-in-life [Accessed March 2023]

UKHSA (2023): Guidance on the hepatitis B antenatal screening and selective neonatal immunisation pathway https://www.gov.uk/government/publications/hepatitis-b-antenatal-screening-and-selective-neonatal-immunisation-pathway/guidance-on-the-hepatitis-b-antenatal-screening-and-selective-neonatal-immunisation-pathway%2D%2D2 [Accessed August 2024]

UKHSA Annual Flu Programme (online) https://www.gov.uk/government/collections/annual-flu-programme

UKHSA (2023) Flu vaccination programme 2022 to 2023: information for healthcare practitioners https://www.gov.uk/government/publications/flu-vaccination-programme-information-for-healthcare-practitioners [Accessed March 2023]

UKHSA (2024a): Pertussis (whooping cough) vaccination programme for pregnant women: information for healthcare practitioners https://www.gov.uk/government/publications/vaccination-against-pertussis-whooping-cough-for-pregnant-women/pertussis-whooping-cough-vaccination-programme-for-pregnant-women [Accessed August 2024]

UKHSA (2024b). Confirmed cases of pertussis in England by month. https://www.gov.uk/government/publications/pertussis-epidemiology-in-england-2024/confirmed-cases-of-pertussis-in-england-by-month (accessed May 2024)

UKHSA (2024c) RSV vaccination of pregnant women for infant protection: information for healthcare practitioners RSV vaccination of pregnant women for infant protection: information for healthcare practitioners - GOV.UK (www.gov.uk) [Accessed August 2024]

UKHSA (on line): Immunisation against infectious diseases (The Green Book) (on Line) https://www.gov.uk/government/collections/immunisation-against-infectious-disease-the-green-book

UKHSA (on line): Immunisation against infectious diseases (The Green Book) (on Line) Rubella Chapter 28 https://www.gov.uk/government/publications/rubella-the-green-book-chapter-28

UKHSA (on line): Immunisation against infectious diseases (The Green Book) (on Line) RSV Chapter 27a https://www.gov.uk/government/publications/respiratory-syncytial-virus-the-green-book-chapter-27a

UKHSA (2023) Hepatitis B: guidance, data and analysis vaccination and Hepatitis B: guidance, data and analysis. https://www.gov.uk/government/collections/hepatitis-b-guidance-data-and-analysis#infants-born-to-hepatitis-b-infected-mothers

UKHSA (2021): Changing the timing of the neonatal BCG immunisation programme to a 28 day immunisation programme: effective from 1 September 2021 https://www.gov.uk/government/publications/bcg-vaccine-information-on-the-28-day-immunisation-programme/changing-the-timing-of-the-neonatal-bcg-immunisation-programme-to-a-28-day-immunisation-programme-effective-from-1-september-2021

UKHSA (2021a): BCG vaccination and SCID screening: patient pathway https://www.gov.uk/government/publications/bcg-vaccination-and-scid-screening-patient-pathway

UKHSA (2021b): The safety of COVID-19 vaccines when given in pregnancy. Available at: The safety of COVID-19 vaccines when given in pregnancy - GOV.UK (www.gov.uk) [Accessed March 2023].

UKHSA, 2022a. COVID-19 vaccination programme. Information for healthcare practitioners. Available at: COVID-19 vaccine information for healthcare practitioners (publishing.service.gov.uk) Accessed March 2023.

Vishram et al (2017) Vaccination in pregnancy: Attitudes of nurses, midwives and health visitors in England. https://www.ncbi.nlm.nih.gov/pubmed/29048989 [Accessed March 2023]

WHO (2024) Maternal and Neonatal Tetanus Elimination (MNTE) https://www.who.int/initiatives/maternal-and-neonatal-tetanus-elimination-(mnte) (accessed May 2024)

2.2 Section 2: Vaccine Preventable Disease in Infancy and Early Childhood

Helen Bedford

Abstract

This section considers vaccines for infants and children. The early years are an important time of life for vaccination, with the largest number of vaccines across the life course offered in the first 5 years. Babies and young children are at risk of severe infections, and timely vaccination is important to provide protection against a series of significant diseases.

This section discusses aspects of the development of the routine vaccination schedule for young children over the past 30 years.

Detailed information of the specific programmes is available in the Green Book and guidance for healthcare professionals.

2.2.1 Introduction

The first 5 years of life is the most active period for vaccination throughout the life course. In the UK in 2024, vaccines against 14 diseases are offered routinely, most requiring multiple doses. The rationale for this is clear—infants and young children are at high risk of severe disease from many infections, and to maximise the preventive benefits of vaccines, it is vital to protect them before they reach the peak age for an attack. For example, the peak age for an attack of meningococcal group B infection is 5 months of age (Public Health England 2021). For some vaccines, there is a balance between vaccinating too early and ensuring a good immune response, for example, measles vaccine; persistence of measles antibodies acquired prenatally from an immune mother can neutralize the live attenuated vaccine virus interfering with the infant's ability to mount a strong immune response (Manikkavasagan and Ramsay 2009). Vaccine development over the years has meant that UK children can be afforded protection against an increasing number of potentially serious infections causing illness, complications or even death.

In this section, the evolution of the UK childhood vaccination programme will be discussed. Although not a full account (for this, see Lang et al. 2020a and Lang et al. 2020b), some key developments will be highlighted and the rationale for the frequent changes to the vaccine schedule explained. Detailed explanation for each vaccine is available in the relevant Green Book chapter and associated guidance for healthcare professionals. It is important that vaccinators are aware of the changes to the schedule over time, so they can discuss these issues if raised.

2.2.2 Key Stages in the Development of the UK Routine Childhood Vaccination Programme

In UK, the comprehensive vaccine schedule for children aged under 5 years has developed over many years. See the UK **Routine childhood immunisation schedule Routine childhood immunisation schedule—GOV.UK**.

The following are examples of these changes:

- In 1987, only five vaccines—diphtheria, tetanus, pertussis (whole cell), oral polio and measles—were offered routinely for young children. The timing of doses was spaced out with doses at 3 months, 4.5–5 months and 8.5–11 months—single measles vaccine was offered at 12–18 months and a booster of diphtheria, tetanus (DT) and polio at 4–5 years (DHSS 1988). Diphtheria, tetanus and pertussis were available in combinations of diphtheria, tetanus and pertussis (DTP) or diphtheria and tetanus (DT) with oral polio (OPV) given at the same time. Because of the existing availability of a pertussis free combination (DT), many parents declined DPT following controversy over the safety of whole cell pertussis vaccine starting in the 1970s; this vaccine safety scare resulted in very poor uptake (30%) of pertussis vaccine for several years followed by three large outbreaks of disease and many deaths (Baker 2003). This is an important example

of the impact of providing choice about vaccine formulations which can undermine vaccine confidence.
- In 1990, the timing of the primary course was accelerated with diphtheria, tetanus and pertussis vaccine offered at 8, 12 and 16 weeks. The aim of this was to enable earlier protection (particularly to pertussis) and, with precise ages for administration rather than the previous age ranges, to facilitate timely vaccination and increase uptake. As attendance at clinics tends to decline in children over the age of 6 months, as parents return to work, it was hoped that the accelerated schedule would result in improved vaccine uptake (Lang et al 2019b).
- In 2004, acellular pertussis vaccine replaced the whole cell pertussis vaccine as it causes fewer side effects such as fever and irritability. At the same time, inactivated injectable polio vaccine replaced the live oral vaccine—this was in line with WHO advice to switch to inactivated polio to avoid the risk of vaccine associated paralytic polio. Although very rare, this posed a greater risk than that of natural infection which had been eliminated from the UK with the last case acquired in the UK in 1984 (UKHSA 2023).
- To facilitate administration and maximise cost effectiveness and uptake, there has been an expansion in the number of vaccines included in combination over the past two decades. For example, at the time of writing, a "6-in-1" vaccine containing DTaP/IPV/Hib/HepB is routinely used for the primary vaccine course in the UK.
- The combined measles, mumps and rubella (MMR) vaccine offered at 12–18 months was introduced in 1988 replacing the single antigen measles vaccine. In 1996, the timing of MMR vaccine was tightened to 12–15 months and a second dose introduced at 3–5 years (DHSS 1996) to ensure the 5–10% of vaccinees who do not develop immunity to the measles component after one dose of MMR vaccine develop protection.

The development of the UK vaccine schedule over 30 years from the late 1980s has resulted from the changing epidemiology of vaccine preventable diseases due to vaccination, availability of new vaccines, new formulations of vaccines and the accumulation of evidence about vaccine effectiveness and of safety and cost effectiveness.

2.2.3 Improvements in Vaccine Uptake

Between 1979 and 1990, vaccine uptake improved considerably from 80 to 89% for diphtheria, tetanus and polio, from 51 to 84% for measles and from 35 to 78% for pertussis. These improvements were reported to be due to a combination of organisational change, health education and professional commitment to the programme (White et al 1992). There was also variation in rates from 40 to 95% between health districts (Begg and White 1988). Current vaccine uptake is discussed further in Chaps. 6 and 12.

2.2.4 Case Study of Meningococcal C Vaccine

This case study, in Box 2.1, highlights how vaccine programmes respond to changes in epidemiology of an infection and accumulating information about vaccine effectiveness. Although vaccine trials are often large, it sometimes requires vaccines to be used at a population level for some years to develop in-depth understanding of vaccine effectiveness. The introduction of meningococcal C vaccine provides an example of how vaccine policy has changed over the years as evidence has accumulated about the vaccine's effectiveness and meningococcal C disease has become uncommon.

> **Box 2.1 Introduction and Evolution of the UK Meningococcal C Vaccine Programme**
>
> A vaccine to protect against meningococcal group C infection was introduced in the UK, the first country to introduce the vaccine in 1999.
>
> The 1990s saw an increase in cases of all meningococcal infections in England and Wales with a particular increase in cases of group C disease among adolescents caused by a very virulent strain with a high case fatality—this was mirrored in other countries (Campbell et al. 2009).
>
> The increase in cases triggered a vaccine research programme to gather the necessary information about the safety and immunogenicity of meningococcal C conjugate vaccines. A Hib conjugate vaccine introduced in 1992 had already proven successful in reducing Hib disease in the UK. The first Men C conjugate vaccine was licensed in the UK in September 1999, and a vaccine programme was introduced on November 1, 1999, for 2-, 3- and 4-month-olds with a catch-up campaign for all children and young people aged 4 months to 17 years—this was later increased to 24 years.
>
> With high uptake of the vaccine, disease rates reduced. This was not only in the cohorts who received the vaccine but also the wider population. The vaccine does not only provide direct protection, but by reducing asymptomatic nasopharyngeal carriage of the organism, it also provides indirect protection leading to community (herd) protection.
>
> Evidence showed that although the vaccine given in infancy was effective, effectiveness declined rapidly from a year after the last dose. In 2006, a booster dose of MenC vaccine (Hib/MenC) was introduced at 12 months of age to maintain immunity through the childhood years. As it became evident that fewer doses of MenC vaccine in infancy were adequate to provide immunity, and the disease became very uncommon in young children, the number of doses of vaccine recommended in infancy was reduced from three to none between 2006 and 2016 (Campbell et al 2009; PHE 2014; PHE 2016). As nasopharyngeal carriage of MenC peaks in the teenage years, a teenage dose of vaccine was introduced in 2013/2014 (PHE 2016). From 2015, this was offered as MenACWY vaccine.

(continued)

> **Box 2.1** (continued)
>
> The meningococcal C vaccine programme has been highly successful with a 99% reduction in cases from 1999 to 2024 and only three cases reported between July 2023 and June 2024; two of these three cases occurred in adults older than 25 years (UKHSA 2024a). In view of this excellent control of MenC disease, the focus for future maintenance of herd immunity is teenagers. The discontinuation of Hib/MenC vaccine at 12 months in 2025 leaves the teenage dose of MenACWY vaccine as the only dose of MenC which will be given to continue to maintain community immunity (Department of Health and Social Care 2022).

2.2.5 Selective Vaccines for Infants and Young Children

Young age, some health conditions or other factors place children at higher risk of either acquiring an infection, for example, tuberculosis, hepatitis B and influenza, or being more severely affected if they catch it, such as influenza and tuberculosis.

2.2.5.1 Hepatitis B Vaccine

Babies born to women who are chronic carriers of hepatitis B virus or who had an acute hepatitis B infection in pregnancy are at high risk of becoming chronic carriers of the infection due to perinatal transmission of the virus. This chronic carriage can result in liver cancer or cirrhosis in later life (see section on vaccination in pregnancy and neonates in Chap. 2). Universal antenatal screening for hepatitis B has been recommended in the UK since 1998 (Giraudon et al 2009) with babies born to infected mothers offered a four-dose hepatitis B vaccination course and immunoglobulin (depending how infectious the mother is). However, districts performed differently in ensuring at risk babies received all four doses of vaccine, with less than half of all at risk babies in London not completing the vaccination course in 2006 (Giraudon et al 2009). Since 2017, hepatitis B vaccine has been offered routinely to all UK babies as part of the routine schedule, with high-risk infants given additional doses of the vaccine at birth, 4 weeks and 12 months (Green Book 2024) (note: as part of a number of changes to the UK vaccine schedule, from 2025 the 12 month dose will be discontinued).

2.2.5.2 Influenza Vaccine

Influenza is often perceived by parents to be less serious than other vaccine preventable infections (UKHSA 2024b). However, influenza infection rates are not only higher in pre-school and school aged children than in adults, but hospitalisation rates are highest among children under 5 years of age and children with chronic health conditions who are particularly at risk of severe disease (Boddington et al 2021). In England between 2015 and 2020, there was an average of 40 deaths every year from flu among children under 4 years of age (PHE 2020).

In addition to the routine schedule, influenza vaccine is recommended for people with chronic health conditions aged 6 months onward. However, uptake of the vaccine in the 6-month to 2-year age group is very poor. In 2022–2023 GP data showed this did not exceed 25% for any of the risk groups (UKHSA 2023).

2.2.5.3 BCG Vaccine

The UK has a low tuberculosis (TB) incidence (7.75 per 100,000 in 2022), with rates higher in some urban areas, e.g. London. Rates are also highest among people born outside the UK and in socially deprived groups (UKHSA 2022). The BCG vaccine has been in use in the UK for over 70 years with changes to the schedule over the years as the epidemiology of TB changed. At first offered universally to all school leavers (aged 14), the vaccine is now offered selectively. The main group offered BCG are babies with an increased risk of being in contact with TB. BCG is offered to babies to protect them against the more severe forms of the disease such as TB meningitis. Such babies are those whose parents or grandparents were born in countries with an incidence of TB of 40 per 100,000 or higher (UKHSA 2022) or living in areas of England where the annual TB incidence is 40/100,000 or higher. The vaccine is offered by 28 days after birth or soon after. BCG is also offered to older children and adults if needed.

2.2.6 Vaccination of Premature Infants

Premature infants are at increased risk of infection. For example, studies have found that premature infants are at higher risk of invasive meningococcal disease and of poorer outcome from the disease (Calvert et al 2024). This increased risk of infection persists beyond the perinatal period into childhood, and so it is particularly important that they receive all the recommended vaccines in the routine schedule at the recommended chronological age (Angelidou and Levy 2020). Although there is evidence that premature infants may not produce such a strong immune response as full term infants, there is usually high enough production of antibodies to provide short term protection which is boosted by further doses. For further details, see the relevant Green Book chapter.

2.2.7 Summary

The early years represent the period when most vaccines in the UK schedule are offered. This is to provide protection when babies and children are at greatest risk of catching certain infections and most vulnerable to their severe consequences. The UK schedule has developed over the past 30 years to include many more vaccines and as a result has become more complex. Vaccine programmes are under constant review resulting in frequent changes to the schedule. It is important that vaccinators are able to discuss the reasons for such changes with parents and patients to maintain vaccine confidence.

References

Angelidou, A. and Levy, O., 2020. Vaccination of term and preterm infants. Neoreviews, 21(12), pp.e817-e827.

Baker, J.P., 2003. The pertussis vaccine controversy in Great Britain, 1974–1986. Vaccine, 21(25-26), pp.4003-4010.

Begg, N.T. and White, J.M., 1988. A survey of pre-school vaccination programmes in England and Wales. Journal of Public Health, 10(4), pp.344-350.

Boddington, N.L., Pearson, I., Whitaker, H., Mangtani, P. and Pebody, R.G., 2021. Effectiveness of influenza vaccination in preventing hospitalization due to influenza in children: a systematic review and meta-analysis. Clinical Infectious Diseases, 73(9), pp.1722-1732.

Calvert, A., Campbell, H., Heath, P.T., Jones, C.E., Le Doare, K., Mensah, A. and Ladhani, S., 2024, April. Risk of Invasive Meningococcal Disease in Preterm Infants. In *Open Forum Infectious Diseases* (Vol. 11, No. 4, p. ofae164). US: Oxford University Press.

Campbell, H., Borrow, R., Salisbury, D. and Miller, E., 2009. Meningococcal C conjugate vaccine: the experience in England and Wales. Vaccine, 27, pp. B20-B29.

Department of Health and Social Security, Welsh Office, Scottish Home and Health Department. Immunisation against Infectious Disease HMSO 1988 https://wellcomecollection.org/works/ahmwg6w9/items

Department of Health 1996. Immunisation against Infectious disease. Eds DM Salisbury and NT Begg. HMSO.

Giraudon, I., Forde, J., Maguire, H., Arnold, J. and Permalloo, N., 2009. Antenatal screening and prevalence of infection: surveillance in London, 2000-2007. Eurosurveillance, 14(9), p.19134.

Lang S, Loving S, McCarthy ND, et al Two centuries of immunisation in the UK (part I). Archives of Disease in Childhood 2020a;105:115-121.

Lang S, Loving S, McCarthy ND, et al Two centuries of immunisation in the UK (part II). Archives of Disease in Childhood 2020b;105:216-222.

Manikkavasagan, G. and Ramsay, M., 2009. Protecting infants against measles in England and Wales: a review. Archives of disease in childhood, 94(9), pp.681-685.

Public Health England 2014. Changes to the meningococcal C conjugate (MenC) vaccine schedule 2013-2015 https://assets.publishing.service.gov.uk/media/5a7d5996ed915d28e9f39c1f/MenC_information_for_healthcare_professionals_V7_.pdf

Public Health England 2016. Removal of the infant dose of meningococcal serogroup C (MenC) conjugate vaccine given at three months from 1 July 2016. https://assets.publishing.service.gov.uk/media/5a80300de5274a2e8ab4eb1e/2016_MenC_infant_schedule_letter-FINAL__1_.pdf

Public Health England. Surveillance of Influenza and other respiratory viruses in the UK Winter 2019-2020. https://webarchive.nationalarchives.gov.uk/ukgwa/20220401215804/https:/www.gov.uk/government/statistics/annual-flu-reports

Public Health England 2021. Meningococcal B vaccination: Information for healthcare practitioners. https://assets.publishing.service.gov.uk/media/60ddb1fdd3bf7f7c2ed84ba7/Meningococcal_B_vaccination_information_for_healthcare_practitioners_July21.pdf

UKHSA 2023 Green book Chapter 26 Poliomyelitis https://assets.publishing.service.gov.uk/media/5a7a084140f0b66a2fbff665/Green-Book-Chapter-26-Polio-updated-18-January-2013.pdf

UKHSA 2024. Tuberculosis in England, 2023 report https://www.gov.uk/government/publications/tuberculosis-in-england-2023-report-data-up-to-end-of-2022/tb-incidence-and-epidemiology-england-2022

UKHSA 2022. Vaccine Update: issue 327, April 2022m SCID, TB and BCG special edition. https://www.gov.uk/government/publications/vaccine-update-issue-327-may-2022-scid-tb-and-bcg-special-edition/vaccine-update-issue-327-april-2022-scid-tb-and-bcg-special-edition

Department of Health and Social Care 2022. Joint Committee on vaccination and Immunisation (JCVI) interim statement on the Immunisation schedule for children. https://www.gov.uk/government/publications/jcvi-interim-statement-on-changes-to-the-childhood-immunisation-schedule/joint-committee-on-vaccination-and-immunisation-jcvi-interim-statement-on-the-immunisation-schedule-for-children

UKHSA 2023. Seasonal Influenza Vaccine uptake in GP patients. https://assets.publishing.service.gov.uk/media/64d21e33a4045e000da84be5/GP-patients-flu-annual-report-2022-2023.pdf

UKHSA 2024a. Invasive meningococcal disease in England: annual laboratory confirmed reports for epidemiological years 2023 to 2024. https://www.gov.uk/government/publications/meningococcal-disease-laboratory-confirmed-cases-in-england-2023-to-2024/invasive-meningococcal-disease-in-england-annual-laboratory-confirmed-reports-for-epidemiological-year-2023-to-2024

UKHSA 2024b. Childhood vaccines: parental attitudes survey 2023 findings. https://www.gov.uk/government/publications/childhood-vaccines-parental-attitudes-survey-2023/childhood-vaccines-parental-attitudes-survey-2023-findings

White, J.M., Gillam, S.J., Begg, N.T. and Farrington, C.P., 1992. Vaccine coverage: recent trends and future prospects. *British Medical Journal*, *304*(6828), pp.682-684.

2.3 Section 3: Vaccine Preventable Disease in Older Children and Young People

Michelle Falconer[1], Helen Eley[2], Emma Adamson[3]
[1] Public Health Scotland, London, UK
[2] Design, Implementation and Clinical Guidance Division, UK Health Security Agency, London, UK
[3] London, UK

Abstract
This section focuses on the importance of vaccination to control infectious disease in children (over the age of 5 years) and young people.

Ensuring children and young people have easy access to vaccinations is crucial. For older children and young people, going to the GP surgery for vaccine appointments can become an unnecessary barrier; offering vaccinations in schools during school hours is an effective strategy to overcome the difficulties of attending the GP.

Keywords: Access of vaccines for older children and young people

- HPV vaccine
- MMR
- Tailoring vaccine programmes

2.3.1 Introduction

Increasingly, the UK routine vaccination schedule offers vaccines throughout people's lives. Older children and young people (CYP) require vaccination to protect them against potentially life-threatening disease which may be because of their age, e.g. approaching or reaching their sexual debut and becoming eligible for HPV vaccine, or because of an increased risk of exposure to some vaccine preventable diseases due to their educational, travel or career choices (Falconer, 2017). Other situations when vaccines may be required include catching up with previous missed doses to complete a course (e.g. MMR) or the routine offer of a booster dose (e.g. Td/IPV).

Research published by the Royal Society for Public Health (RSPH) found that although there were variations according to ethnic background, most CYP trust vaccines and think they are important for their health. However, there was also a reported lack of awareness about the vaccines available to them with just over half of the participants aware of HPV (52%) and meningitis (57%) vaccines, but, despite being eligible for the vaccines, only 39% knew this was the case (Aguilar *et al.*, 2023).

RSPH also identified several factors that would encourage CYP to have a vaccine. Although receiving information about vaccines from trusted sources was rated highly (71%), more than half of the CYP reported that being able to have a vaccine at school (53%) or near their home (55%) would encourage them to have it (Aguilar P et al, 2023) supporting the current school-based vaccination strategy.

As schools are places of daily attendance, they provide a convenient setting to offer vaccinations to CYP. Vaccinating in the school setting can help to achieve higher vaccine coverage, enable CYP to seek support from their peers and school nurses during the vaccination procedure and may help to promote a positive vaccination experience. However, as not all school aged children attend school, such as those who are home educated or who have been excluded from school, consideration also needs to be given to ensuring they are not disadvantaged by not being able to complete the recommended schedule.

Partnerships within local healthcare systems such as integrated care systems (ICSs) and health boards (HBs) are crucial to ensure a whole system approach is taken to address inequalities in vaccination uptake. This should include using local intelligence and vaccine uptake data to target resources and interventions to increase uptake. An example of how this may work in a local area is described in Box 2.2 where the local team again worked with the local Iman to support uptake of the influenza vaccine among the Muslim community.

> **Box 2.2 Example Case Study for Tailoring Immunisation Programmes: Influenza**
> The Sirona School Aged Immunisation Team runs flu vaccination clinics at mosques across Bristol to improve accessibility for children from the Muslim community to receive the injectable vaccine.
>
> This was organised following feedback from a parent from the Bristol Muslim community after his child was unable to receive the nasal flu vaccine in school for religious reasons, due to its porcine gelatine content.
>
> The School Aged Immunisation Team contacted him to see if he would be able to facilitate a flu clinic at his Mosque. The clinic was arranged, advertised and promoted within the community and the event was well attended. The team now work collaboratively with three Mosques within BNSSG, delivering both the injectable flu vaccine and also offering MMR catch up vaccinations.
>
> During the 2024/2025 flu campaign over 200 vaccines were delivered in Mosque settings to school aged children and their younger siblings. Building on the success of this we are now offering intramuscular (IM) flu vaccination at secondary schools, special schools and some after school clinics at primary schools where we know there is a high demand.
>
> *Example provided by Alix Towson Lead for School Aged Immunisations—Sirona CIC Bristol*

Other community leaders could similarly be involved in the provision of tailored messages that are delivered in languages understood by parents/carers and influential members of communities to address any myths and misconceptions (Maravia, 2023).

2.3.2 The National Routine Childhood Immunisation Schedule

2.3.2.1 Rationale for Vaccination in CYP

The national routine child and adolescent immunisation schedule (UKHSA, 2024) recommends vaccines for school aged children and young people through to 18 years of age.

These include influenza vaccine offered annually, HPV vaccine, meningococcal ACWY vaccine and a booster of tetanus, diphtheria and polio vaccines. These vaccine appointments also provide an opportunity to check young people are up to date with the remainder of the schedule. Individuals' risk of infection may change with changing epidemiology. For example, the introduction of the quadrivalent meningococcal ACWY vaccine followed a significant increase in the incidence of meningococcal W disease in older teenagers and young adults (UKHSA/DHSC, 2022). It is recognised that while asymptomatic carriage of meningococcal bacteria occurs in around 10% of the population, carriage rates increase in older teenager and young adults making vaccination in this age group particularly important to reduce transmission to the rest of the population (Christensen et al. 2010).

Since vaccination during the school day happens without a parent being present, there are a number of considerations for successful vaccination.

2.3.2.2 Consent *(Covered in Detail in Chap. 7 in the Book)*

Consent to vaccinate is normally obtained from parents in advance. If CYP attend for vaccination without parental consent, the capacity of the CYP to provide self-consent will need to be assessed. Fisher et al. (2019) explored barriers and enablers to adolescent self-consent for vaccination. They suggested that the policy context in place for delivery of vaccination governs the implementation of adolescent self-consent procedures and that "a desire to protect the reputation of professionals and the role of parents in decision-making" is also hindering the implementation of self-consent procedures for adolescents.

As the provision of informed consent is a key requirement before any vaccination can proceed regardless of age, supporting young people to understand health interventions such as vaccination and encouraging them to make responsible decisions and then to self-consent can help to develop their health literacy and their confidence.

2.3.2.3 Preparation for Vaccination

During or after vaccination, CYP may experience anxiety or fainting. The Centers for Disease Control and Prevention (CDC, US, 2005) reported that fainting after vaccination is common in adolescents, and one study of vaccine adverse events reported that 62% of syncope events occurred in adolescents 11–18 years old.

It is also important to acknowledge that CYP's fear and concerns about pain associated with injections and of adverse reactions can be a significant barrier to vaccination (Tadio et al 2022).

The vaccination team will be required to acknowledge any anxieties, reassure CYP, manage any fainting episodes and respond confidently to any anxiety induced events to ensure a positive vaccination experience and that they recognise the benefits of future vaccination, not only for their own future health, for example, when travelling, but also for their own children, if and when they become parents.

The details of each recommended vaccine and their impact on the diseases they are preventing are available in the Green Book—see Box 2.3 for the HPV vaccine.

> **Box 2.3 HPV vaccine**
> The human papillomavirus (HPV) vaccine has been offered to all girls in the UK since 2008 and from September 2019 routinely offered to all teenagers, girls and boys universally, as they are approaching or reaching their sexual debut. It is also offered to men who have sex with men.
>
> HPV is predominantly sexually transmitted but essentially spread by close contact, and most unvaccinated people will get it at some point in their lives. Most infections will not cause symptoms and will resolve completely on their own; some, however, will develop into cancer and genital warts. The vaccine helps to protect against cervical cancer, some cancers of the head and neck and some anogenital cancers. More than 280 million doses of the HPV vaccine have been given worldwide, including 120 million doses in the USA and over 10 million in the UK.
>
> The vaccine has proved highly successful—it has reduced HPV infections and cervical cancer rates in vaccinated cohorts (Falcaro et al. 2021, 2024). A reduction in precancerous lesions and evidence of herd protection have also been observed in unvaccinated individuals (Kavanagh *et al,*. 2017). This success offers real hope that cervical cancer could be eliminated (defined as fewer than 4 cases per 100,000; Gultekin et al. 2020) although this will require continued high vaccination coverage.
>
> Full details of the UK vaccine programme are available in the Green Book "HPV" chapter.

See Box 2.4 for MMR.

School vaccination clinics provide a continued opportunity to receive the vaccines required to ensure young people are fully protected against specific diseases. School vaccination also provides an opportunity to inform young people about infectious diseases, healthy lifestyle options and how by having vaccines they are not only protecting themselves but helping to prevent infection spreading to others in the community.

> **Box 2.4 MMR Vaccine**
> There was a significant fall in the uptake of the MMR vaccine in the early 2000s due to parental concerns about vaccine safety following publication of the now discredited paper suggesting a link between the vaccine and autism.
> Based on data from 2014 to 2016, the UK achieved WHO measles elimination status, (defined as the absence of circulating measles in the presence of high vaccine coverage) (PHE 2019). However, subsequently, the combination of a decline in vaccine uptake in the UK (NHS Digital) and large numbers of unvaccinated people who have accumulated over two decades has allowed measles to take hold once more with a large outbreak over 2023/2024 (UKHSA 2024a), demonstrating the need for sustained high vaccine uptake.
> Mumps infections have also risen (UKHSA, 2022). Although some of this may be due to the protection against the mumps component of the vaccine waning over time, young people and adults aged 15 and over who missed out on MMR vaccine when they were younger have been particularly affected by both measles and mumps infections. Two doses of MMR vaccine are required to achieve lasting protection. For those currently unvaccinated or partially vaccinated (i.e. only had one dose of MMR vaccine) catch up of any missed doses is recommended regardless of time since first dose.
> Rubella is now very uncommon in the UK, however, rare cases of congenital rubella have occurred in babies of unvaccinated mothers, not born in the UK (UKHSA 2024b). Young people who have not received two doses of MMR vaccine remain susceptible to rubella and may be at risk of infection when travelling. It is therefore important to remind everyone of the importance of catching up with missed MMR doses.
> *The 'Green Book', chapter 21—Measles, chapter 23—Mumps and chapter 28—Rubella provides full details on the MMR vaccine programme*

2.3.3 Conclusion

Vaccinating CYP at key stages in their lives is a core part of the UK vaccination programme. As new vaccines are introduced, it can be challenging ensuring high uptake. However, for most young people, a compulsory element of growing up is having access to an educational setting. School-based vaccination provision is invaluable to ensure unimmunised or partially immunised CYP have the opportunity to catch up. See Box 2.5 for key issues to consider.

> **Box 2.5 Summary and Key Messages**
> - Every opportunity should be used to vaccinate and to catch up CYP who are not fully immunised.
> - Routinely checking vaccination status when children start or change schools is a good opportunity to remind parents and students of any doses needed to complete a course.
> - Addressing barriers to immunisation (including reducing anxiety in CYP and ensuring opportunities for self-consent are in place where appropriate/required) can help to facilitate high vaccine coverage.
> - Young people have reported that they are encouraged to take up the offer of a vaccine if it is available near to their home or school.
> - Systems should be available to increase awareness in young people of recommended vaccines, the diseases that they protect against and why they are recommended. This could be through access to websites, social media platforms, reminder services and social media pop ups.
> - Working with system partners to address parents'/carers' misconceptions may help to improve uptake of vaccines.

References

Aguilar Perez F, Ramsey R, Satherley P, Vohra J. (2023) RSPH: Children and Young People's attitudes towards vaccinations – what they know and what they have to say [Online]. March 2023. Available at: https://www.rsph.org.uk/our-work/policy/vaccinations/children-and-young-adults-attitudes-towards-vaccinations-what-they-know-and-what-they-have-to-say.html

Christensen H, May M, Bowen L, Hickman M, Trotter C L, (2010) Meningococcal carriage by age: a systematic review and meta-analysis Lancet: https://doi.org/10.1016/S1473-3099(10)70251-6 (accessed 13th June 2023)

Falcaro M, Castañon A, Ndlela B, Checchi M, Soldan K, Lopez-Bernal J, Elliss-Brookes L, Sasieni P (2021). The effects of the national HPV vaccination programme in England, UK, on cervical cancer and grade 3 cervical intraepithelial neoplasia incidence: a register-based observational study. *Lancet* 298(10316).

Falcaro M, Soldan K, Ndlela B, Sasieni P. Effect of the HPV vaccination programme on incidence of cervical cancer and grade 3 cervical intraepithelial neoplasia by socioeconomic deprivation in England: population based observational study. BMJ. 2024 May 15;385:e077341. https://doi.org/10.1136/bmj-2023-077341. PMID: 38749552; PMCID: PMC11094700.

Falconer M (2017): *Improving vaccine coverage in adolescence and beyond* Available at: https://www.tandfonline.com/doi/full/10.1080/21645515.2017.1394535 (Accessed: 08 June 2023)

Fisher, H., Harding, S., Hickman, M., Macleod, J., & Audrey, S. (2019). Barriers and enablers to adolescent self-consent for vaccination: A mixed-methods evidence synthesis. Vaccine, 37(3), 417-429. https://doi.org/10.1016/j.vaccine.2018.12.007

Gov.UK (2018) Measles outbreaks across England Available at: https://www.gov.uk/government/news/measles-outbreaks-across-england Accessed on: 09 June 2023

Gultekin et al (2023) *World Health Organization call for action to eliminate cervical cancer globally* International journal of gynaecological cancer Available at World Health Organization call for action to eliminate cervical cancer globally | International Journal of Gynecologic Cancer (bmj.com) Accessed 08 June 2023)

JCVI (2018) Statement on HPV vaccination Joint Committee on Vaccination and Immunisation Available at: https://www.gov.uk/government/publications/jcvi-statement-extending-the-hpv-vaccination-programme-conclusions Accessed on: 09 June 2023

Kavanagh K, Pollock KG, Cuschieri K, Palmer T, Cameron RL, Watt C, Bhatia R, Moore C, Cubie H, Cruickshank M, Robertson C. Changes in the prevalence of human papillomavirus following a national bivalent human papillomavirus vaccination programme in Scotland: a 7-year cross-sectional study. Lancet Infect Dis. 2017 Dec;17(12):1293-1302. https://doi.org/10.1016/S1473-3099(17)30468-1. Epub 2017 Sep 28. PMID: 28965955.

NHS Digital Childhood Vaccination statistics published annually https://digital.nhs.uk/data-and-information/publications/statistical/nhs-immunisation-statistics (Accessed November 2024)

Maravia U, (2023) *HPV Vaccines: Clinical assistance to sin or prevent STIs?* Journal of the British Islamic Medical Association Available at: Microsoft Word - 2_Ethics 3_ Usman (jbima.com) Accessed: 08 June 2023

MMWR Syncope after vaccination – United States, January 2005 – 2007 Available at: Syncope After Vaccination --- United States, January 2005--July 2007 (cdc.gov) Accessed: 08 June 2023

NHS (2022) A guide to immunisation for young people Available at: https://www.gov.uk/government/publications/immunisations-for-young-people Accessed: 09 June 2023

PHE 2019. UK Measles and Rubella elimination strategy 2019.https://assets.publishing.service.gov.uk/media/5c35e849ed915d732cade0a5/UK_measles_and_rubella_elimination_strategy.pdf

Taddio, A., McMurtry, C.M., Logeman, C., Gudzak, V., de Boer, A., Constantin, K., Lee, S., Moline, R., Uleryk, E., Chera, T. and MacDonald, N.E., (2022). Prevalence of pain and fear as barriers to vaccination in children–Systematic review and meta-analysis. *Vaccine*, 40(52), pp.7526-7537.

UKHSA (2023). Complete routine immunisation schedule. Available at https://www.gov.uk/government/publications/the-complete-routine-immunisation-schedule Accessed: April 2024

UKHSA (2019) Measles in England Available at: https://publichealthmatters.blog.gov.uk/2019/08/19/measles-in-england/ Accessed on: 09 June 2023

UKHSA, (2022) Mumps: notifications and confirmed cases by oral fluid testing in England, 2013to 2022 by quarter Available at: Mumps: notifications and confirmed cases by oral fluid testing in England, 2013 to 2022 by quarter - GOV.UK (www.gov.uk) (Accessed on: November 2024)

UKHSA (online) Immunisation against infectious disease (the Green book), Measles (chapter 21), available at Measles: the green book, chapter 21 - GOV.UK (www.gov.uk) Accessed 09 June 2023

UKHSA (online) Immunisation against infectious disease (the Green book), Human Papillomavirus (HPV) (chapter 18a), available at Green Book HPV chapter 18a (publishing.service.gov.uk) Accessed 09 June 2023

UKHSA (online) Immunisation against infectious disease (the Green book), Influenza (chapter 19), available at Influenza: the green book, chapter 19 - GOV.UK (www.gov.uk) https://www.gov.uk/government/publications/measles-the-green-book-chapter-21 Accessed 09 June 2023

UKHSA (online) Immunisation against infectious disease (the Green book), meningococcal (chapter 22), available at Meningococcal: the green book, chapter 22 - GOV.UK (www.gov.uk) Accessed: 09 June 2023

UKHSA, (2024a) Latest measles epidemiology published Measles epidemiology 2023 and 2024 - GOV.UK (www.gov.uk) [November 2024)

UKHSA (2024b) Laboratory confirmed cases of measles, rubella and mumps in England: October to December 2023 https://www.gov.uk/government/publications/measles-mumps-and-rubella-lab-confirmed-cases-in-england-2023.

2.4 Section 4: Vaccine Preventable Disease in Adults

Helen Donovan
London, UK

> **Abstract**
> This section focuses on the importance of vaccination to control infectious disease at all stages of life and particularly in people as they age and are at increased risk due to having chronic health conditions or because of their occupation.
> The section will consider specifically the following:
>
> - Vaccination throughout life
> - Occupational health
> - Tetanus vaccination
> - Immunosenescence
> - Specific vaccines given to older adults

2.4.1 Introduction

Most vaccines are given to infants and children and are recommended as early as possible in the life course. For many vaccines, however, it is never too late to catch up on any missed in childhood. It should be an underlying principle to ensure that adults have had the full course of all the routine vaccines.

However, adults are at increased risk of severe illness and more serious consequences from some infections. This might be because of increasing age which leads individuals to become less able to cope with infections due to immunosenescence (described below). Underlying medical conditions may mean people are at greater risk of more significant sequelae from the disease. For some people, their likelihood of exposure to an infection is increased due to lifestyle or occupation. As a result, specific vaccines are recommended for adults.

2.4.2 Vaccination Throughout Life

People remain eligible throughout their lives for vaccines against a range of infections including tetanus, diphtheria, polio, measles, mumps and rubella. It is essential that people who missed out on vaccination as children or who are migrants to the country, including adults, are offered the vaccines they are eligible for. Opportunities to ensure they are fully vaccinated or reminded about the importance of vaccination should be taken, for example, in adolescence, when travelling or during pregnancy (see the relevant sections in this chapter on adolescence, travel and vaccines in pregnancy)—also see Box 2.6, "Key vaccines recommended for all".

> **Box 2.6 Key Vaccines Recommended for All**
> **Tetanus**: Tetanus vaccination was introduced routinely in the UK in 1961 although many people in the armed forces will have had the vaccine from the 1930s or as ad hoc boosters at other stages in their lives. However, they may not have had a full five dose course of vaccine; cases of tetanus are still reported, predominantly in under-vaccinated adults over the age of 64 years (UKHSA 2023).
> **Tetanus: the Green Book, Chapter 30**
> **Diphtheria**: It is now very rare in the UK following the introduction of routine vaccination in 1942. However, cases have gradually increased over the last 10 years. This is in part due to enhanced surveillance and testing, but a significant number of cases have been in migrants coming to the UK as asylum seekers and generally in those who have not been fully immunised (UKHSA 2023a).
> **Diphtheria: the Green Book, Chapter 15**
> **Polio**: Vaccination has almost eradicated polio disease with only two countries in the world where wild polio virus remains endemic (Global Polio Eradication Initiative on line). Only when wild polio is eradicated from a country and there is no risk of imported wild polio virus can the live oral polio vaccine (OPV) be completely replaced by the inactivated polio vaccine (IPV)—countries where polio remains endemic use a combined OPV/IPV schedule. Recently vaccinated (with live polio vaccine) individuals excrete the live polio virus, and it has the potential to mutate and cause vaccine derived polio disease (VDPD). This is an ongoing challenge for the UK population and across the world with unvaccinated people remaining at risk (UKHSA 2023b).
> **Polio: the Green Book, Chapter 26**
> Nurses should take opportunities to check the immunisation status of adults. Where appropriate, vaccination should be offered based on the guidance in the UKHSA "Vaccination of individuals with uncertain or incomplete immunisation status" algorithm (UKHSA online). The UKHSA migrant health guide also provides information and resources for those coming to the country on the vaccines they are entitled to (OHID 2021).

Vaccination provides essential safeguards and protections for people at all stages of life. It is important that the messaging around vaccination focuses on the positive benefits for overall health and wellbeing across the life course and to be encouraged as part and parcel of healthy life choices (Doherty et al. 2019). As with all vaccine programmes, a high uptake across the eligible population is needed. The World Health Organization has also promoted the role of vaccination in the prevention and control of antimicrobial resistance (WHO 2021).

It is forecast that by 2045, 4.3% of the UK population will be 85 years or older (ONS 2022). This brings with it an associated increase in age-related diseases, a higher susceptibility to infections and other conditions (WHO 2022). Furthermore, the ONS report (2022) projects that the UK population will also increase as a result of net migration.

The details of each vaccine programme are available in the Green Book.

The UKHSA "Vaccination of individuals with uncertain or incomplete immunisation status" (UKHSA online) provides guidance on the recommended vaccines in infancy and childhood and from age 10 through to adulthood, as shown in Fig. 2.1.

Additional vaccines are required for some occupations (see below). Further information is available in the Green Book Chap. 12 "Immunisation of Healthcare and Laboratory Staff".

Some medical conditions increase the risk of complications from infectious diseases—they can weaken the immune system and make recovery harder. Individuals with long-term conditions may require additional vaccines or additional doses of vaccines to provide better protection—Chap. 7 in the Green Book, "Immunisation of Individuals with Underlying Medical Conditions", details which vaccines and when they should be given alongside the specific disease chapters.

2.4.3 Immunosenescence

Immunosenescence describes a range of changes that occur in all components of the immune system and results in loss of immune function with a decreased capacity to respond to infections and vaccines as we age (Crooke et al. 2019). With ageing, the immune system's response to vaccines in the production of antibodies or as immune memory is lower compared to that of younger people. Different vaccine technologies and strategies may be required to boost the vaccine response, for example:

- Vaccines with adjuvants or higher dose concentrations, such as the influenza vaccines
- Different delivery systems to administer the vaccines, such as using intradermal or transcutaneous routes
- Repeated booster doses, for example, for the COVID-19 vaccines

2.4.4 Vaccine Accessibility

Vaccination services must be easily available with consideration given to how to improve accessibility for all. Some groups may be at particular risk of severe disease, for example, the very elderly and those identified with learning disability were considerably impacted by the COVID-19 pandemic (ONS 2021 and PHE 2020). People who are physically frail or who have cognitive impairment or learning difficulties may need specific consideration from the service; those with the greatest

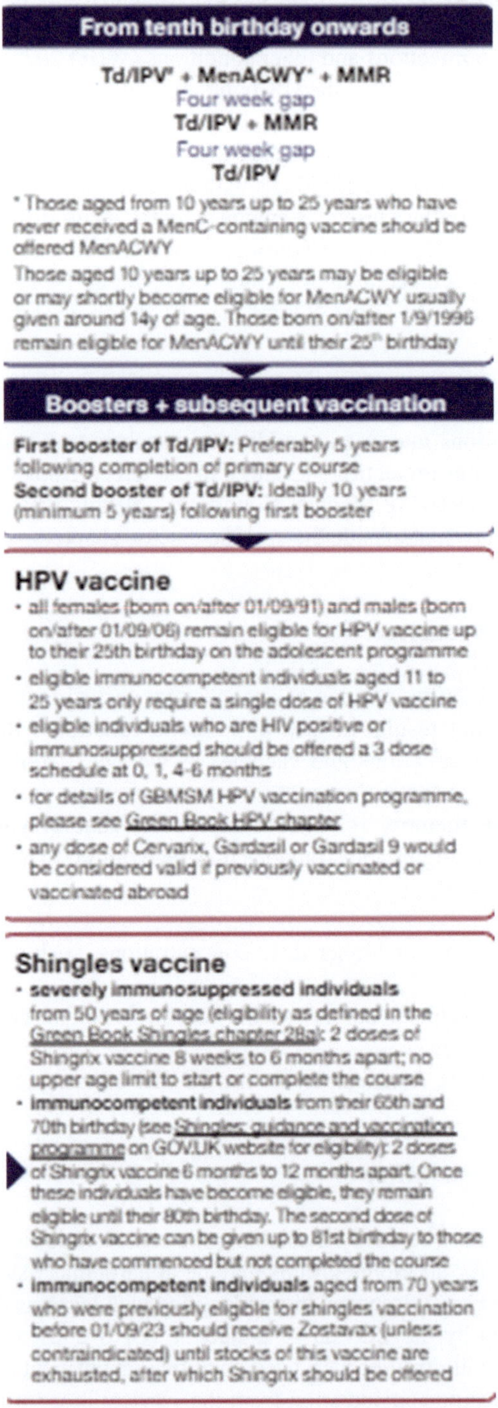

From tenth birthday onwards

Td/IPV* + MenACWY* + MMR
Four week gap
Td/IPV + MMR
Four week gap
Td/IPV

* Those aged from 10 years up to 25 years who have never received a MenC-containing vaccine should be offered MenACWY

Those aged 10 years up to 25 years may be eligible or may shortly become eligible for MenACWY usually given around 14y of age. Those born on/after 1/9/1996 remain eligible for MenACWY until their 25th birthday

Boosters + subsequent vaccination

First booster of Td/IPV: Preferably 5 years following completion of primary course
Second booster of Td/IPV: Ideally 10 years (minimum 5 years) following first booster

HPV vaccine

- all females (born on/after 01/09/91) and males (born on/after 01/09/06) remain eligible for HPV vaccine up to their 25th birthday on the adolescent programme
- eligible immunocompetent individuals aged 11 to 25 years only require a single dose of HPV vaccine
- eligible individuals who are HIV positive or immunosuppressed should be offered a 3 dose schedule at 0, 1, 4-6 months
- for details of GBMSM HPV vaccination programme, please see Green Book HPV chapter
- any dose of Cervarix, Gardasil or Gardasil 9 would be considered valid if previously vaccinated or vaccinated abroad

Shingles vaccine

- **severely immunosuppressed individuals** from 50 years of age (eligibility as defined in the Green Book Shingles chapter 28a): 2 doses of Shingrix vaccine 8 weeks to 6 months apart; no upper age limit to start or complete the course
- **immunocompetent individuals** from their 65th and 70th birthday (see Shingles: guidance and vaccination programme on GOV.UK website for eligibility): 2 doses of Shingrix vaccine 6 months to 12 months apart. Once these individuals have become eligible, they remain eligible until their 80th birthday. The second dose of Shingrix vaccine can be given up to 81st birthday to those who have commenced but not completed the course
- **immunocompetent individuals** aged from 70 years who were previously eligible for shingles vaccination before 01/09/23 should receive Zostavax (unless contraindicated) until stocks of this vaccine are exhausted, after which Shingrix should be offered

Fig. 2.1 UKHSA vaccination of individuals with uncertain or incomplete immunisation. Image showing vaccines recommended for all those 10 years and older. The resource is updated regularly (UKHSA online)

access difficulties are indeed the most likely to need vaccination. Chapter 7 on consent also discusses the principles for making a "best interest" decision where an individual is unable to consent to having a vaccine.

There are steps immunisers should consider ensuring the service is accessible to everyone. Chapter 10 considers these and the clinic management in detail.

2.4.5 Vaccines for Occupational Health

Vaccines are also recommended for certain occupational groups to help protect them and the vulnerable people they work with. It is beyond the scope of this book to list all the occupations where specific or additional vaccines are recommended, but they include healthcare workers, laboratory workers and environmental health officers. Occupational health vaccine requirements vary depending on the occupation and the specific disease risks they may be exposed to throughout their employment but will generally include ensuring workers are fully up to date with vaccines in the national schedule and offering some additional vaccines, such as hepatitis, rabies, tuberculosis and chickenpox, depending on the area of work.

The Green Book Chap. 12 "Immunisation of Healthcare and Laboratory Staff" (UKHSA online), and the individual disease chapters, provides the specific details of any vaccines required and the rationale for this. It also details the recommended schedule and any pre-employment and ongoing vaccination or testing necessary for the individual's particular role and work.

2.4.6 Specific Vaccines Recommended for Adults

The following provides an overview of some vaccines that are currently routinely recommended in the UK for older adults and those with underlying comorbidities or immunosuppression. The programmes are complex, and the details for each vary considerably depending on the burden of the specific vaccine preventable disease—they are all detailed in the Green Book (UKHSA online) and specific guidance for healthcare professionals.

Influenza: Influenza "flu" infection for many people is self-limiting, but for those with other underlying conditions, who are immunosuppressed, the young or elderly, it can be life threatening.

Influenza vaccine is routinely recommended, on an annual basis, for older adults (generally over 65 years) and those with underlying health conditions. Influenza: the Green Book, Chapter 19

Pneumococcal disease: It covers several conditions caused by the bacterium *Streptococcus pneumoniae* (also known as the pneumococcus) including invasive pneumococcal meningitis, pneumonia and pneumococcal septicaemia. There are over 90 different serotypes of this bacterium which can be carried in the nasal passages with no symptoms but transmitted to others causing illness. The disease particularly affects the very young, under 1 year of age, older adults over 65 years of age and those with underlying medical conditions.

The vaccination programme has been successful in controlling infection caused by the pneumococcal serotypes contained in the vaccines. However, infection with non-vaccine serotypes continues to be prevalent in the population with some increasing as a result of serotype replacement; new vaccines providing more effective protection against a wider spectrum of serotypes are in development.

Alongside the routine children's vaccine programme, pneumococcal vaccine is also recommended for older adults and those with underlying medical conditions. Pneumococcal: the Green Book, Chapter 25

Shingles: Shingles or *herpes zoster* is a viral infection which develops from a reactivation of latent varicella zoster virus (VZV). Most adults in the UK have been exposed to VZV, and on recovery from chickenpox disease, the virus lies dormant in the dorsal nerve cells and can reactivate as people get older or where the immune system is compromised (UKHSA 2022).

The shingles vaccine programme aims to reduce the incidence and severity of shingles disease in adults, in whom the risk of severe disease and of subsequent post herpetic neuralgia (PHN) is higher. Shingles (herpes zoster): the Green Book, Chapter 28a

Respiratory syncytial virus (RSV): Over the last few years, there have been vaccine options developed for respiratory syncytial virus (RSV), a common virus which causes cold like symptoms. While the main burden of disease is in infants and children under 5, it can also cause respiratory illness in the elderly and those living with frailty and comorbidities. The full impact of respiratory syncytial virus (RSV) as people get older is probably underestimated; however, the Green Book advises that prior to vaccination, RSV has been estimated to account for 175,000 annual GP episodes in those aged 65 years and older in the UK. It is estimated that there are 4,000 deaths due to RSV in those aged over 75 years in England and Wales. As such, an RSV vaccine programme to reduce the incidence and severity of RSV disease in older people has been introduced from September 2024 following JCVI recommendation (JCVI 2023). The RSV vaccine should be offered to all individuals 75 years and over with a catch-up programme implemented for those up to 80 years of age (UKHSA 2024). There is a separate programme to vaccinate pregnant women designed to protect infants (see the section on vaccines in pregnancy in this chapter).

It is also important to consider the COVID-19 vaccines which are not, as yet, part of the routine vaccination programme. Older adults and those with underlying health conditions have been offered regular boosters for COVID-19 over the last few years dependent on their age and/or increased risk of severe infection due to underlying conditions; this is likely to evolve. See also the section on vaccines for emerging public health threats.

2.4.7 Conclusion

Vaccination throughout adult life is a core part of the UK vaccination programme. It is inevitable that more vaccines will be introduced and different strategies for improving acceptance of vaccines will be developed as a contribution to healthy ageing. Further research on immunosenescence, how this affects vaccination in older people and how new vaccines help to tackle this will be needed. Box 2.7 gives a summary and key messages.

> **Box 2.7 Key Messages**
> - Vaccination throughout life has a key role as part of wider preventive public health interventions.
> - A greater focus on the vaccination of older adults is important due to immunosenescence, antimicrobial resistance and global migration.
>   - Ensure all adults are up to date with the routine vaccination schedule with vaccines against tetanus, diphtheria, polio and measles, mumps and rubella.
>   - Adults in certain occupational groups will require additional vaccines to protect them and the populations they work with.
>   - Adults with other health conditions will need additional vaccines.
>   - All adults over the age of 65 are recommended one dose of pneumococcal vaccine.
>   - All adults over the age of 65 are recommended an annual influenza vaccine.
>   - All adults identified in the programme for the shingles vaccine should have generally two doses as soon as they become eligible.
>
> The specific chapters in the Green Book relating to these infections contain more detail.

References

Crooke SN, Ovsyannikova IG, Poland GA, Kennedy RB. (2019): Immunosenescence: A systems-level overview of immune cell biology and strategies for improving vaccine responses. Experimental Gerontology Volume 124

Doherty M T, Del Giudice G and Maggi S. (2019) Adult vaccination as part of a healthy lifestyle: moving from medical intervention to health promotion Annuls of Medicine Published on line 2019 Apr 26. https://doi.org/10.1080/0785389 0.2019.1588470 (accessed June 2023)

JCVI (2023) Independent report Respiratory syncytial virus (RSV) immunisation programme for infants and older adults: JCVI full statement, 11 September 2023 https://www.gov.uk/government/publications/rsv-immunisation-programme-jcvi-advice-7-june-2023/respiratory-syncytial-virus-rsv-immunisation-programme-for-infants-and-older-adults-jcvi-full-statement-11-september-2023

OHID (2021) Immunisation: migrant health guide Immunisation: migrant health guide - GOV.UK (www.gov.uk) (accessed June 2023)

ONS (2021) Deaths from COVID-19 by age band https://www.ons.gov.uk/aboutus/transparencyandgovernance/freedomofinformationfoi/deathsfromcovid19byageband (accessed June 2023)

ONS (2022) National population projections: 2020-based interim National population projections - Office for National Statistics (accessed June 2023)

Pera A, Campos C, López N, Hassouneh F, Alonso C, Tarazona R, Solana R (2015): Immunosenescence: Implications for response to infection and vaccination in older people. J.*maturitas* 82(1):50-5.

UKHSA (online) Immunisation against infectious disease – 'The Green Book' available on line https://www.gov.uk/government/collections/immunisation-against-infectious-disease-the-green-book

UKHSA (on line) Vaccination of individuals with uncertain or incomplete immunisation status https://www.gov.uk/government/publications/vaccination-of-individuals-with-uncertain-or-incomplete-immunisation-status (last accessed July 2025)

UKHSA (2022) Vaccination against Shingles Information for healthcare professionals https://www.gov.uk/government/publications/shingles-vaccination-guidance-for-healthcare-professionals

UKHSA (2023a) Diphtheria in England: annual reports 2022 updated May 2023 https://www.gov.uk/government/publications/diphtheria-in-england-and-wales-annual-reports/diphtheria-in-england-2022

UKHSA (2023b) Polio immunisation response in London 2022 to 2023: information for healthcare practitioners Polio immunisation response in London 2022 to 2023: information for healthcare practitioners - GOV.UK (www.gov.uk)

UKHSA (on line): Immunisation against infectious diseases (The Green Book) (on Line) RSV Chapter 27a https://www.gov.uk/government/publications/respiratory-syncytial-virus-the-green-book-chapter-27a

UKHSA (2024): RSV vaccination of older adults: information for healthcare practitioners https://www.gov.uk/government/publications/respiratory-syncytial-virus-rsv-programme-information-for-healthcare-professionals/rsv-vaccination-of-older-adults-information-for-healthcare-practioners

PHE now UKHSA (2019) Tetanus Guidance on the management of suspected tetanus cases and on the assessment and management of tetanus-prone wounds https://www.gov.uk/government/publications/tetanus-advice-for-health-professionals

WHO (2022) Ageing and health https://www.who.int/news-room/fact-sheets/detail/ageing-and-health

WHO 2021 Leveraging Vaccines to Reduce Antibiotic Use and Prevent Antimicrobial Resistance (who.int) (accessed June 2023)

2.5 Section 5: Vaccine Preventable Diseases in Travellers and Traveller Vaccines

Sandra Grieve

> **Abstract**
> This section will look at the specific vaccine preventable travel-related diseases and their management from a travel health perspective.
> For each disease, vaccinators should also consult the National Travel Health Network and Centre (NaTHNaC) fact sheet and the Green Book chapter.
> The US Centers for Disease Control (CDC) yellow book is also recommended to provide the international perspective.
> UK guidance should always be followed when advising and recommending vaccines for travellers from the UK.
> Keywords: Travel health and travel vaccines

2.5.1 Introduction

Travel health (TH) is a specialist field of practice which can be challenging. In the UK, TH services are mainly delivered by registered nurses, predominately in a primary care setting but also in pharmacies and private travel clinics. Travel abroad may expose travellers to diseases not present in the UK. Pretravel consultations provide an ideal opportunity to ensure that individuals are up to date with their routine UK vaccines. The SARS-CoV-2 pandemic highlighted how quickly diseases can spread around the globe resulting in disrupted international travel and interrupted immunisation programmes globally. The knock-on impact continues to affect the risk of exposure to many diseases such as measles and polio for travellers visiting some destinations. When vaccination rates decline, these diseases may re-emerge so careful advice and prevention guidance are paramount.

This section will look at the specific vaccine preventable travel-related diseases. Current UK and country of practice guidance should always be followed.

2.5.2 Risk Assessment

Nurses should understand the concept of a pretravel risk assessment as the first step in identifying a traveller's potential risks, vaccine recommendations and other travel health requirements. People of all ages travel for a variety of reasons, so focus is always on the individual. The assessment entails collecting information about the traveller and their trip, including a medical and vaccine history and review of age-appropriate routine immunisations. Advice should incorporate personal protection measures for diseases which are not vaccine preventable, e.g. malaria. Some vaccines may be given earlier than the UK recommended schedule for international travel (RCN 2023), for example, MMR given to infants under a year. The UK population is diverse, travelling internationally for a variety of reasons, mainly for leisure. Travellers may not have previously received all the vaccines recommended in the routine immunisation schedule—where appropriate, these should be advised alongside any specifically recommended for travel. The WHO and ECDC provide information on country specific vaccination programmes (WHO, ECDC).

Before or during the pretravel consultation, a tailored questionnaire can be completed by the individual to aid the risk assessment and identify risks, vaccine availability and make sure the appropriate medicines authorisation is available in advance such as having a Patient Specific Direction (PSD), (see Chap. 8). Questionnaire examples can be found in the RCN competencies or on the NaTHNaC website and adapted if necessary. The person conducting the assessment should ensure that questions are understood and answered correctly. Travellers with additional needs may require shared care with another medical specialist, for example, those with long-term conditions or immunosuppression. This can take time but is crucial for the traveller's health and safety. Accurate records should be documented on the computer system, or in an online form, including discussions, consent and any vaccine refusals (RCN 2023).

Settled migrants returning to their country of origin to visit friends and relatives (VFRs) present a different risk profile to holidaymakers. They often stay longer, live closely with the local population, may not seek pretravel advice and often underestimate their health risks. As the rate of imported disease can be higher in this group, advice and vaccinations are particularly important (OHID 2021). Evidence-based national resources are available online for practitioners and the public (NaTHNaC, TRAVAX, Fitfortravel).

Following the assessment and identification of potential disease risks, recommendations on vaccine preventable diseases can be discussed and vaccines and advice offered as appropriate. Vaccine schedules may be determined by the time available, but even if departure is imminent, it is usually possible to offer advice and some vaccine protection. Travellers should be reminded of the importance of completing vaccine schedules, which may involve arranging appointments to complete courses overseas or on return. Comprehensive travel insurance is essential for all travellers.

2.5.3 Travel Health Services

Nurses should follow age-appropriate national immunisation schedules, taking into account their workplace setting and individual UK country differences regarding travel vaccine recommendations (Green Book). Depending on the service provider, some vaccines for travel are given under NHS provision while others are not.

Confusion arises in the category where vaccines can be given as either an NHS or private service. It's important that any routine vaccines for which people are eligible, including vaccines for travel, should be available to them through NHS services. For nurses in GP settings, a policy must be in place as to which vaccines are an NHS provision and which are entirely private. Services should be clearly defined and not mixed (BMA). Those providing travel health services should familiarise themselves with the guidance.

2.5.4 Vaccines for Travel

Not every travel-related disease is vaccine preventable. Vaccines can be categorised as follows:

- Routine—childhood and adult according to national schedule
- Recommended—according to risk
- Required—for crossing international borders

It is beyond the scope of this chapter to provide detail on every vaccine requirement for the traveller. This requires a careful history of the precise travel itinerary, any occupational or lifestyle risks and the potential risk of exposure for the individual. This needs to be considered alongside an understanding of the disease prevalence rates and endemicity in the country(s) being visited and before vaccine recommendations are provided alongside other relevant health advice, e.g. malaria.

The specific disease chapters in the Green Book provide the details for each vaccine, the infections and exact vaccination recommendations and requirements from a travel perspective.

Table 2.1 provides a summary of some of the specific vaccine preventable diseases where vaccines may be recommended or required before travel and grouped against how the disease is transmitted:

- Through the faecal-oral route
- Through contact with infected bodily fluids
- Through close association with infected individuals
- Via transmission from mosquitos and other vectors
- Via transmission from animals (zoonotic transmission)

Box 2.8 summarises the key messages.

Table 2.1 Vaccine preventable disease where travel vaccines may be recommended categorised according to route of transmission. *For further information for the specific disease and vaccines, see the relevant chapters in the Green Book online or the section for the disease on the National Travel Health Networks and Centre (NaTHNaC) website*

Disease transmission: faecal-oral route
Cholera
Is considered a disease of poverty, associated with lack of sanitation and clean water. It is endemic in many areas of Asia and Africa and is contracted by ingesting contaminated food or water
Most travellers are at low risk but those living or working in resource-poor conditions, e.g. aid relief workers, are at greater risk
General advice on good hygiene precautions and self-treatment of diarrhoea
Vaccination is recommended for adults and children from age 2 years who are assessed to be at risk
Hepatitis A virus (HAV)
Is found worldwide although prevalence varies. It is generally higher in low-income countries, where sanitary conditions are poor or where infrastructure is damaged, e.g. during natural disasters. It is also contracted through direct contact
Travel abroad is a common factor in imported cases and UK travellers are unlikely to be immune. Long-stay travellers, VFRs or aid workers are at higher risk. It is one of the most common travel-related vaccine preventable diseases and highly transmissible
General advice on personal and food hygiene. High-starred hotels do not guarantee protection as hygiene may be poor
Vaccination is recommended for travellers, including those at occupational or lifestyle risk, visiting areas of high or intermediate prevalence
Polio
Transmitted through food and water contaminated by human faeces in areas of poor sanitation and hygiene
Polio is on the verge of global eradication but remains endemic in two countries: Afghanistan and Pakistan. Until poliovirus transmission is interrupted, all countries remain at risk of importation. Countries with low oral polio virus (OPV) coverage in routine immunisation programmes also risk cases and outbreaks caused by circulating vaccine-derived poliovirus (cVDPVs)
Polio is rare in UK travellers, but risk is increased if visiting areas reporting outbreaks or cVDPV, e.g. long-stay healthcare or aid workers working in areas of poor hygiene. A Public Health Emergency of International Concern (PHEIC) was declared in 2014 and remains in place under continual review, putting temporary recommendations in place for travellers (WHO 2024)
Vaccination through the UK routine schedule provides a minimum of five doses. Based on their travel plans, activities and medical history, additional doses may be required for travel, to prevent global spread. Travellers to areas or countries reporting recent polio cases may need an additional booster dose, and those visiting certain countries for over 4 weeks may be required to show proof of vaccination 4 weeks–12 months before leaving that country (Green Book)

(continued)

Table 2.1 (continued)

Typhoid/paratyphoid
These enteric fevers are acquired by ingesting food or water contaminated by *Salmonella* Typhi and *Salmonella* Paratyphi A, B or C. Previous exposure does not confer immunity. Low-income countries with lack of access to safe food, water and sanitation pose a risk
Most imported cases in England and Wales are in those visiting friends and relatives (VFRs) who travelled to India, Pakistan and Bangladesh
Strict food, water and hygiene precautions, especially before meals, are essential. Enteric fever can be treated with antibiotics but drug-resistant and extensively drug-resistant (XDR) strains are being reported. Such cases have been seen in returned UK travellers, emphasising the importance of advising and vaccinating travellers visiting risk areas
Vaccination is recommended according to individual risk, e.g. travel to the Indian subcontinent
Disease transmission: blood and bodily fluids
Hepatitis B virus (HBV)
Is transmitted by contact with the blood or bodily fluids of an infected person. HBV causes subclinical, acute and chronic disease and can be fatal. It is found worldwide—risk is higher in, e.g. the Western Pacific, East Asia and sub-Saharan Africa
For most travellers, the risk is low but related to destination, endemicity and lifestyle. Exposure can be reduced by awareness and behaviour, e.g. avoiding unprotected sex, skin piercing, tattoos or sharing drug injecting equipment
UK travellers visiting areas of high or intermediate prevalence who place themselves at risk abroad should be offered immunisation. Contact sports and undergoing medical or dental procedures in countries with unsafe medical practice pose a risk. Accidents are common abroad—emergency treatment with potentially contaminated medical equipment in resource-poor countries increases risk. Sexual transmission is an important consideration for travellers to Asia
Vaccination is now routine in the UK schedule since 2017 but older children and adults may be recommended vaccine according to individual risk
Disease transmission: contact close association with infected individuals
COVID-19
Caused by SARS-CoV-2 and transmitted primarily through respiratory droplets and aerosols and from direct person-to-person contact. COVID-19 cases are reported worldwide and most countries present a potential risk to travellers. Travellers should ensure they access current FCDO advice and destination requirements before departure and be prepared for changes to guidance at any point (FCDO 2024)
All travellers, particularly those at higher risk of severe COVID-19 infection, should consider their personal risk of infection before travel and ensure they are up to date with the recommended UK COVID-19 vaccines and any seasonal boosters. Proof of vaccination may be requested at any time during the trip (NaTHNaC COVID-19)
The usual personal protection and hygiene measures should be maintained abroad. Travellers should have comprehensive travel insurance which includes repatriation
Meningococcal disease
Meningococcal disease occurs worldwide, with the highest incidence in the "meningitis belt" of sub-Saharan Africa. The risk is increased in travellers visiting countries within the meningitis belt or during an outbreak. Those staying long term, in crowded accommodation or in close contact with local populations heighten risk of exposure. Due to the sudden onset and quick progression of disease, travellers visiting remote areas with limited access to healthcare are at increased risk
Some meningococcal vaccines form part of the UK routine schedule. Vaccination is recommended for pilgrims or seasonal workers travelling to Hajj or Umrah who may live closely with local populations or be in crowded conditions and close contact with people from countries with higher rates of disease—vaccine requirements are posted annually

(continued)

Table 2.1 (continued)

Disease transmission: mosquitos
Dengue
Dengue is a mosquito-borne disease caused by a *Flavivirus and* transmitted by the bite of an infected *Aedes* spp. mosquito
There are four distinct serotypes of dengue virus—DEN 1, DEN 2, DEN 3 and DEN 4—each of which can cause dengue or severe dengue (dengue haemorrhagic fever (DHF)). Dengue occurs in tropical and sub-tropical climates worldwide and is an emerging disease outside of tropical areas, including in Europe. The number of reported cases is increasing in UK travellers, mostly acquired in Asia, the Americas and the Caribbean. Human-to-human transmission has been reported in parts of Asia and Africa, where jungle primates act as a reservoir for the virus. All travellers to dengue endemic countries are at risk particularly during mosquito feeding time between dawn and dusk
Dengue cases are rising globally. Travellers should be advised of dengue at the destination and vigilance on mosquito bite prevention. Vaccination can be considered for those over 4 years who have proof of **dengue infection in the past** and plan to travel to risk areas or areas with an ongoing dengue outbreak. A careful risk assessment is essential (NaTHNaC 2024)
Japanese encephalitis (JE)
Is a mosquito-borne flavivirus infection transmitted to humans from pigs and wading birds via the bite of an infected *Culex* spp. mosquito, mainly in rural Southeast Asia and the Indian subcontinent where rice cultivation and pig farming are common. There is no human-to-human transmission
Traveller's risk is low but increased with prolonged stays in areas where JE is known to occur, e.g. one month or longer in rural areas. Rural outdoor or night-time activities increase risk
Travellers to JE endemic areas should be advised of the seriousness of the disease and mosquito bite prevention measures
Vaccination is recommended for travellers to endemic areas
Yellow fever (YF)
Is an acute viral haemorrhagic disease caused by a flavivirus circulating between infected monkeys or humans and mosquitoes and transmitted through the bite of an infected mosquito (commonly *Aedes aegypti,* more active by day). YF is found in tropical Africa, Central and South America and Trinidad (Caribbean). Infection severity varies, from a mild flu-like illness to severe haemorrhagic disease with a high mortality rate
Under the International Health Regulations (IHR), yellow fever (YF) vaccine is only administered at designated centres (WHO 2005). An International Certificate of Vaccination or Prophylaxis (ICVP), designed to show proof of vaccination and prevent international spread, may be an entry requirement
If vaccination is contraindicated on medical grounds, an exemption certificate can be issued but the traveller should know that if unvaccinated, they remain vulnerable to exposure. Risk assessment will determine individual risk, but vaccination requirement is not always related to the risk of disease in the destination (WHO 2022)
Vaccination is indicated for adults and children from age 9 months requiring primary immunisation for personal protection—to comply with IHR—or both. A single dose of yellow fever vaccine is considered to offer lifelong protection, but some people at continued risk may be eligible for a booster dose (Green Book). Prior to vaccination, the traveller's age and health status should be considered carefully, e.g. infants under 9 months, adults over 60 or those with medical conditions (MHRA 2019). Vaccine contraindications and precautions should be discussed fully with the traveller before administration. A standardised pre-vaccination checklist has been introduced to ensure the yellow fever vaccine is indicated for the intended travel destination and to enable vaccinators to identify existing contraindications or precautions in individuals before vaccination (NaTHNaC 2021)

(continued)

Table 2.1 (continued)

Disease transmission: other zoonotic (animal transmitted) infections
Rabies
Is an acute encephalitis caused by the rabies virus and transmitted through the saliva of an infected mammal by a bite, scratch or lick to broken skin. All warm-blooded mammals, including bats, are susceptible. Rabies is present on all continents, except Antarctica, with over 95% of human deaths in Asia and Africa, caused mostly by dogs
Children are most vulnerable, but all travellers should avoid animal contact. Rabies cases in travellers are rare but not unknown—identifying potentially rabid animals is difficult to determine. Once symptoms appear, rabies is usually fatal but preventable if postexposure treatment (PET) is provided correctly and quickly. Accessing treatment overseas can be difficult, and availability of rabies vaccines and immunoglobulin varies, especially in rural areas
Following potential exposure, travellers should commence immediate wound care, avoid suturing until treatment has begun and seek prompt medical help. Be aware of current UK guidance and access to contacting specialist care
Vaccination. Preexposure rabies vaccination does not remove the need for urgent medical attention and further vaccine doses, following potential exposure. It is recommended for some travellers according to risk, e.g. working with animals or unable to access prompt medical care. Travellers should carry their vaccine record card and produce it if PET needs to be initiated
Tick-borne encephalitis (TBE)
Is a flavivirus infection, present in tick saliva and affecting the central nervous system. It is transmitted rapidly after a bite. Infection is also possible through consuming unpasteurised dairy products from infected animals
It is rare in UK travellers, but incidence is rising, and risk is increased when visiting known TBE areas. TBE exists in many countries spanning central, eastern and northern Europe, across Russia to parts of East Asia. Infection causes a spectrum of disease, from those infected being asymptomatic and having a mild flu-like illness or a potentially life-threatening illness with severe neurological complications
Vaccination is effective at preventing disease and is recommended for those planning outdoor activities in risk areas. To ensure protection before the spring tick season, vaccination should ideally begin during winter

---

Box 2.8 Key Messages
- Providing travel health advice can be challenging.
- Changes and advice can alter quickly—always source current guidance.
- A comprehensive risk assessment for the individual traveller is essential and forms the basis for advice offered and appropriate vaccinations recommended.
- Be aware of your competence level when providing advice to travellers.
- Long-stay and VFR travellers present a different profile to holidaymakers and often don't seek advice. Imported disease is higher in this group.
- Incidence of diseases in the destination and traveller's medical history and proposed activity(s) guide recommendations.
- Not all travel-related diseases are vaccine preventable.
- Expert help with complex scenarios is available

2.5.5 Conclusion

This section has focused on vaccine preventable diseases specifically related to travel abroad. The wider aspects considered throughout the book are also relevant for advising travellers. The travel health consultation presents an ideal opportunity to ensure that the individual is up to date with the UK routine vaccination programme and to complete any omissions in the schedules. Vaccines for travel-related diseases continue to be developed. With vector-borne diseases increasing, new vaccines are becoming available, e.g. to protect against dengue, chikungunya and Zika.

References

British Medical Association (BMA 2022) Travel medication and vaccinations Travel medication and vaccinations (bma.org.uk) [Last accessed 30 June 2024]

European Centre for Disease Control and Prevention. Vaccination Schedules for individual European Countries and specific age groups Vaccination schedules for individual European countries and specific age groups (europa.eu) [Last accessed 30 June 2024]

Fitfortravel Home - Fit for Travel [last accessed 30 June 2024]

Foreign, Commonwealth and Development Office (FCDO) (2024) Foreign travel advice - GOV.UK (www.gov.uk) [Last accessed 30 June 2024]

Immunisation against infectious disease (the Green Book) Immunisation against infectious disease - GOV.UK (www.gov.uk) [Last accessed 30 June 2024]

MHRA (2019) Yellow fever vaccine (Stamaril®) and fatal adverse reactions: extreme caution needed in people who may be immunosuppressed and those 60 years and older. Yellow fever vaccine (Stamaril) and fatal adverse reactions: extreme caution needed in people who may be immunosuppressed and those 60 years and older - GOV.UK (www.gov.uk) [Last accessed 30 June 2024]

MHRA (2021) Yellow fever vaccine (Stamaril®): new pre-vaccination checklist. Yellow fever vaccine (Stamaril): new pre-vaccination checklist - GOV.UK (www.gov.uk) [Last accessed 30 June 2024]

Migrant Health Guide immunisation; Office for Health Improvement and Disparities (2021)

Migrant health guide - GOV.UK (www.gov.uk) [Last accessed 30 June 2024]

NaTHNaC (2024) TravelHealthPro Dengue Fact Sheet. NaTHNaC - Dengue [Last accessed 05/11/2024]

NaTHNaC (2024) Qdenga® dengue vaccine guidance JCVI deliberations. NaTHNaC - Qdenga® dengue vaccine guidance (travelhealthpro.org.uk) [Last accessed 03 July 2024]

NaTHNaC, PHS (2021) Yellow fever vaccine (Stamaril®): pre-vaccination checklist Yellow fever pre-vaccination checklist YELLOW FEVER ZONE (nathnacyfzone.org.uk) [Last accessed 30 June 2024]

NaTHNaC TravelHealthPro https://travelhealthpro.org.uk/ [last accessed 30 June 2024]

NaTHNaC TravelHealthPro country information NaTHNaC - Country List (travelhealthpro.org.uk) [last accessed 30 June 2024]

NaTHNaC TravelHealthPro COVID-19 NaTHNaC - COVID-19 (travelhealthpro.org.uk) [last accessed 03 July 2024]

NaTHNaC TravelHealthPro Polio vaccination certificate. NaTHNaC - Polio vaccination certificate (travelhealthpro.org.uk) [Last accessed 30 June 2024]

NaTHNaC Yellow Fever Zone YELLOW FEVER ZONE (nathnacyfzone.org.uk) [Last accessed 30 June 2024]

Royal College of Nursing (2023) RCN Travel Health Nursing: career and competence development (2023) RCN Travel Health Nursing: career and competence development | Publications | Royal College of Nursing [Last accessed 30 June 2024]

TRAVAX https://www.travax.nhs.uk/ (registration required) [last accessed 30 June 2024]

UK Health Security Agency (2022) UK and international immunisation schedules comparison tool UK and international immunisation schedules comparison tool - GOV.UK (www.gov.uk) [Last accessed 30 June 2024]

World Health Organization (WHO) Immunisation Data. Vaccine schedules WHO Immunization Data portal - Global [Last accessed 30 June 2024]

World Health Organization (WHO) (2005) International Health Regulations. International health regulations (who.int) [Last accessed 30 June 2024]

World Health Organization (WHO) (2022) Country requirements for Yellow fever vaccination. Countries with risk of yellow fever transmission and countries requiring yellow fever vaccination (November 2022) (who.int) [Last accessed 30 June 2024]

World Health Organization (WHO) (2024) Statement of the thirty-eighth Polio IHR Emergency Committee regarding the International Spread of Polio Virus. Statement following the Thirty-eighth Meeting of the IHR Emergency Committee for Polio (who.int) [last accessed 30 June 2024]

2.6 Section 6: Vaccination: Pandemic and Public Health Disease Threats

Helen Donovan, Helen Bedford

> **Abstract**
> Chapter 2 considers the scope and rationale for vaccines recommended across the life course to protect the population from vaccine preventable disease. Other sections include maternity and vaccines given in pregnancy, children's vaccines, adolescent vaccines, adult vaccines and vaccines for travellers.

(continued)

> This section presents a brief overview of how vaccination is used to support the public health measures for infectious disease control in emergency situations such as disease outbreaks, pandemics and emerging infectious diseases.
>
> Vaccination is a key part of pandemic preparedness, for fighting emerging infections and to achieve disease eradication. This may require the development of new vaccines, for example, for Ebola and Zika; the use of existing vaccines, for example, smallpox vaccine to manage Mpox; or ongoing use of polio vaccine.

2.6.1 Introduction

2.6.1.1 Prevention of Disease in the Pre-vaccine Era

Prior to vaccination, pandemics and outbreaks of disease were managed by treating the disease as effectively as possible. This might involve managing individual symptoms together with efforts to minimise the spread of infection by preventing people mixing. For example, at the time of the most significant recorded plague outbreak, "The Black Death", in 1348, in which 50% of the population of Europe died (Izdebski et al 2022), there was little understanding of how and why the infection could spread beyond the home, let alone across other countries. As plague outbreaks continued, there was an inherent understanding of the need to limit exposure to those who were ill—the homes of the infected were marked as a warning not to enter. "Social distancing" burials and disposal of the dead were conducted to limit exposure as far as possible.

2.6.1.2 Prevention of Disease: Vaccination as a Tool

Despite a lack of understanding about disease transmission, it was observed that in general those who recovered or survived infections were unlikely to succumb again, and attempts were made to induce a milder form of a disease to provide protection against more severe version. Variola major (smallpox), a much-feared endemic disease with a fatality rate of one in three, was the main focus of these attempts for centuries. Evidence is available from 200 BCE of rudimentary attempts to provide immunity, using variolation which involves the transfer of small amounts of smallpox material from person to person through the nose or a scratch in the skin. In 1796, Edward Jenner trialled a "vaccine" using the less virulent cowpox virus, heralding the start of global vaccination against smallpox with its ultimate eradication nearly 200 years later in 1980 (WHO 2024a). However, despite significant developments in the understanding of infectious diseases and in vaccine technology since Jenner's time, not least the discovery of germ theory by Pasteur, developing vaccines against some infections has proven challenging. For example, no viable generic vaccine is yet available for HIV despite much research (Esparza 2024). Despite advances in treatment, HIV remains a global public health issue with ongoing transmission and in 2023 alone was responsible for over half a million deaths with over a million new infections (WHO 2024b). Vaccine development programmes are also focused on preparing potential vaccines for future pandemics and for protection against infections such as bubonic plague.

The SARS-CoV-2 pandemic and the rapid introduction of effective vaccines resulted in an unprecedented focus on the value and safety of vaccine programmes. In 2021, the Global Vaccine Alliance (GAVI) warned that to effectively control the COVID-19 pandemic, a global vaccine approach with no one safe until everyone was vaccinated is required, as well as underlining the importance of addressing inequalities to achieve this (Berkley 2021). This message is relevant for all vaccine programmes and a significant part of the United Nations Sustainable Development Goals (SDGs) (United Nations 2025). This includes the importance of providing reliable and consistent information about how vaccines work, their value in preventing serious disease and death and transmission of infection where relevant and the need to boost immunity to maintain protection.

The focus of this section is on vaccination as a tool to support the management of disease—it is beyond the scope or remit of this book to provide other details on the management of infectious disease—these can be obtained via health protection management resources. Figure 2.2 gives a broad overview for defining emerging infectious diseases and outbreaks and the terms pandemic, epidemic and endemic to support understanding.

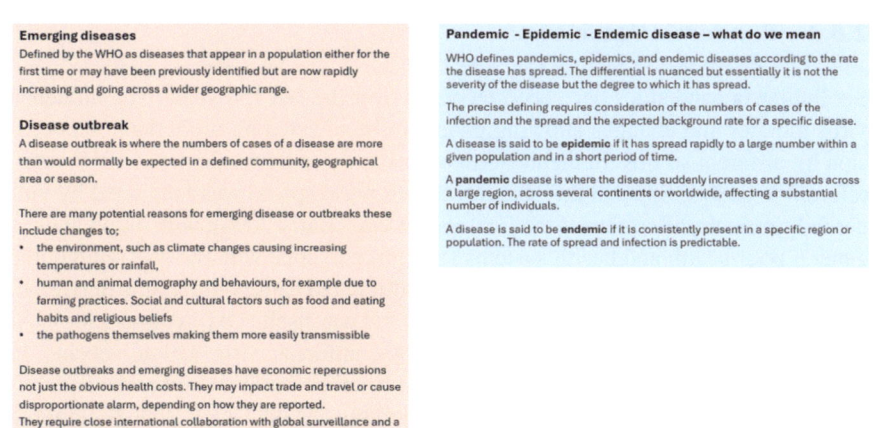

Fig. 2.2 Defining terms (image developed by the authors)

2.6.2 Vaccination in Managing Infectious Disease Outbreaks

The Green Book describes in detail how vaccines work (also referenced in the introduction and value of vaccines). Vaccination alone will not control an outbreak or halt a pandemic, but it provides a significant tool to support the management of such situations. At a basic level, vaccination works in several ways to manage outbreaks and pandemics.

Protecting the individual: Stimulating an immune response so they can fight the infection more effectively (see Chap. 3). Vaccines will not necessarily prevent infection completely but may prevent severe disease. For example, influenza vaccines continue to prevent severe infection and hospitalisation but will not prevent all influenza infections.

Protecting the population: If a vaccine is well matched to the circulating organism and can block infection completely, or enough of the population at greatest risk are vaccinated, there will be far fewer people with severe disease and subsequently fewer people able to pass on infection. This in turn reduces the pressure of the infection on the wider health and care system and wider community. The influenza vaccine given to those at risk of severe disease reduces the numbers needing hospital care.

Preventing transmission and spread of infection: many infections spread between individuals who themselves have no or very mild symptoms. Some vaccines prevent carriage of the organism and so interrupt transmission, such as conjugate vaccines for prevention of meningococcal (MenACWY) and *Haemophilus influenzae* B (Hib) infections.

2.6.3 Pandemic Vaccination

Six influenza pandemics have been recorded over the last 150 years. The influenza virus mutates and changes allowing people to be infected on more than one occasion by different strains. In the most notorious and deadly pandemic in 1918, often referred to as the "Spanish flu", the infection's rapid spread was facilitated by vulnerabilities in the aftermath of the First World War (Barry 2004); with individuals in general poor health and health systems struggling to cope with the war injured, the pandemic is reported to have infected 500 million and caused the deaths of over 40 million people worldwide, more than died in the war itself (Oxford et al 2002) . At the time there was limited understanding of the influenza virus and no vaccine. In the following 100 years, influenza continued to cause seasonal outbreaks and epidemics in addition to further pandemics, notably in 1957 and 1968 (Kilbourne 2006). Although understanding of the different viral strains improved, routine influenza vaccination for high-risk groups only started in the late 1960s, using limited egg-based vaccine technology to develop the vaccine virus.

It wasn't until the 2009 H1N1 "swine flu" pandemic when vaccine technology was sufficiently advanced to enable development of a specific vaccine rapidly; a monovalent H1N1 influenza vaccine was available within 5 months of the outbreak in September 2009. The H1N1 vaccine virus was then incorporated into subsequent seasonal influenza vaccines to manage future waves of the infection. Influenza vaccine technology has developed even further in the last 15 years with different vaccine platforms now available, although the continued evolution of influenza viruses still makes it necessary to vaccinate annually. The risk of other infections leading to significant outbreaks and pandemics remains.

2.6.4 SARS-CoV-2 COVID 19

In late 2019, scientists in China identified a novel coronavirus, SARS CoV2, causing severe respiratory infections and unusual pneumonia. By early January 2020, the Chinese Centers for Disease Control and Prevention shared the genome sequence for SARS-CoV-2 enabling vaccine development (Burki 2023). The SARS-CoV-2 virus spread rapidly causing what became known as COVID-19 disease (CO for corona, VI for virus, DI disease, and 19 for 2019, when the infection was first identified). The World Health Organization (WHO) declared it a pandemic on March 11, 2020 (World Health Organization No date). During 2020, in an attempt to halt transmission and buy time before vaccines became available, countries introduced public health strategies to limit transmission of the virus; travel was limited and other measures included nationwide lockdowns (stay-at-home, school closures, etc.) and social distancing. The impact on education, social interactions and the economy was significant. With scientific collaboration, political will, industrial partnership and public involvement, it was possible to develop, trial and manufacture vaccines to support the pandemic response by the end of 2020.

It is beyond our scope to provide detail of the various SARS-CoV-2 vaccines; those used in the UK programme are described in the Green Book. However, it is important to note that the newer technology of using viral vectors and nucleic acid messenger (mRNA) in the development of COVID vaccines was already well researched and had been considered for vaccines for new and emerging infections such as Zika and Ebola. In Chap. 3, vaccine development more generally is discussed including the process of testing and clinical trials.

The COVID-19 vaccine programme began in the UK in late 2020 (UKHSA 2021) giving the opportunity to manage the infection and enable the world to open up and normal life to resume.

The COVID-19 vaccine programme remains at the forefront of most immunisers' minds; it continues to develop with booster doses recommended for those most at risk. While there are still many COVID-19 infections, vaccination has reduced disease severity. Immunisers across the UK can and should be proud of their significant contribution to this success and continue to ensure those most at risk are offered boosters.

2.6.5 Pandemic Preparedness

The experience of the COVID-19 pandemic, for many a once in a lifetime experience, is focusing political, economic and health leaders to ensure learning informs preparation for future pandemics. Vaccine development and administration is likely to form a central aspect of any future response. Building on the 2021 report from the pandemic preparedness treaty on the 100 Days Mission to Respond to Future Pandemic Threats (House of Commons 2024), the case for collaboration to enable rapid treatment, testing and vaccine development in the first 100 days of future outbreaks and pandemics is clear. The Coalition for Epidemic Preparedness Innovations (CEPI), a global partnership working to accelerate the development of vaccines established after the Ebola disease (EBOD) outbreak in 2014, is working to support the 100 days' aim and helping to identify pathogens to prioritise for vaccine and treatment development. CEPI has identified pathogens such as SARS-CoV-2, EBOD, Lassa fever, MERS-CoV, chikungunya, Nipah and Rift Valley fever viruses as priorities as well as the need to consider as yet unknown novel viral threats with epidemic or pandemic potential, often referred to as "Disease X". In the UK, the UKHSA launched the vaccine development and education centre (VDEC) in 2023 UKHSA's Vaccine Development and Evaluation Centre (VDEC) - GOV.UK with the aim of working with partners and across sectors to enable the development of the vaccines to save lives and mitigate the harm from vaccine preventable disease.

2.6.6 Vaccine Programmes to Manage Disease Outbreaks

Globally, infectious disease patterns are changing with known and emerging infections expanding beyond historical boundaries. Global climatic changes, deforestation, armed conflict and migration and travel are all contributing to opportunities for infections to spread to vulnerable populations and environments with limited experience in disease management. Examples include the 2024 Marburg haemorrhagic disease outbreak in Rwanda (WHO 2024c) and cholera outbreaks in Europe (ECDC 2025). The emergence of locally transmitted cases of dengue in Europe including cases imported to the UK is a cause of significant concern for locals and tourists alike (UKHSA 2024).

There have been significant outbreaks of Ebola and Zika, and, although more localised, increasing globalisation means that an outbreak can quickly spread, requiring global action to manage them. Vaccines against some Ebola strains have been developed using different technologies and used to manage outbreaks and reduce onward transmission (WHO 2020).

There is no vaccine currently for Zika infection although the research is in progress using viral vector technology using adenovirus, similar to the COVID-19 vaccine.

More recently, infections with Mpox have occurred across Europe and America. Although there is no specific Mpox vaccine, the similarity of the virus to smallpox means that new generation smallpox vaccines are effective and have been used successfully as part of the public health management for Mpox (UKHSA 2025).

Polio vaccination has been available since the 1950s and disease eradication a long-term aim for the World Health Organization WHO (GAVI). While no longer a cause of outbreaks, the disease is still a cause for concern, and vaccine programmes remain at the forefront of disease protection. Wild polio remains endemic in only two countries (Pakistan and Afghanistan), and the number of cases is very low, 62 in 2024 (WHO 2024d). The main challenge currently is from the vaccine virus excreted by a recently vaccinated individual which has the potential to mutate, become transmissible and cause infection in others. Most areas in the world have moved to using the inactivated polio vaccine. However, vaccine-derived polio virus was found in sewage in the UK with genetically linked polio virus also found in the USA and Israel, countries previously free of polio. As these countries all have high uptake of polio vaccine and use the inactivated vaccine, this suggests the virus has spread through international travel. There were no cases of polio in the UK, but cases occurred in the USA and in Israel (Hill et al 2022). This emphasises that disease somewhere in the world poses a risk of importations, with vaccination remaining essential until a disease is eradicated/eliminated.

In the UK, the Joint Committee of Vaccination and Immunisation (JCVI) recommended supplementary polio vaccination for those living in high-risk, low vaccine uptake areas and a national drive to ensure the offer of vaccination to all under-vaccinated children.

2.6.7 Conclusion

Vaccines have the potential to significantly weaken the threat of new and emerging pathogens and the devastating impact of epidemics and pandemics. Investment and ongoing international support and partnership are vital to ensure the concerted response required in such situations.

Acknowledgement We would like to thank Professor Sir Andrew Pollard, Director Oxford Vaccine Group and Chair JCVI, for reviewing this section of the chapter.

References

Barry 2004 The site of origin of the 1918 influenza pandemic and its public health implications Journal of Translational Medicine 2004 Jan 20;2:3. https://doi.org/10.1186/1479-5876-2-3

Burki T. (2023) First shared SARS-CoV-2 genome: GISAID vs virological.org. Lancet Microbe. 2023 Jun;4(6): e395. doi: 10.1016/S2666-5247(23)00133-7. Epub 2023 Apr 25. PMID: 37116518; PMCID: PMC10129129.

Berkley S, (2021) No one is safe until everyone is safe. Global Vaccine Alliance GAVI https://www.gavi.org/vaccineswork/no-one-safe-until-everyone-safe

European Centre for Disease Prevention and Control (ECDC) (2025) Cholera worldwide overview

Hill, M., Bandyopadhyay, A.S. and Pollard, A.J., 2022. Emergence of vaccine-derived poliovirus in high-income settings in the absence of oral polio vaccine use. *The Lancet*, *400*(10354), pp.713-715.

House of Commons (2024) What is the proposed WHO Pandemic Preparedness Treaty? – Research briefing https://commonslibrary.parliament.uk/research-briefings/cbp-9550/#:~:text=In%20March%202021%2C%20a%20group,Parliament%20on%2017%20April%202023.

Izdebski, A., Guzowski, P., Poniat, R., Masci, L., Palli, J., Vignola, C., Bauch, M., Cocozza, C., Fernandes, R., Ljungqvist, F.C. and Newfield, T., 2022. Palaeoecological data indicates land-use changes across Europe linked to spatial heterogeneity in mortality during the Black Death pandemic. *Nature ecology & evolution*, *6*(3), pp.297-306. https://www.nature.com/articles/s41559-021-01652-4

Kilbourne, E.D., 2006. Influenza pandemics of the 20th century. *Emerging infectious diseases*, *12*(1), p.9. https://www.ncbi.nlm.nih.gov/pmc/articles/PMC3291411/

Oxford, J.S, Sefton, A, Jackson, R, Innes W, Daniels R.S and Johnson N.P. (2002). World War I may have allowed the emergence of "Spanish" influenza. *The Lancet infectious diseases*. *2*(2), pp.111-114.

United Nations (2025) Department of Economic and Social Affairs Sustainable Development https://sdgs.un.org/

UK Health Security Agency. (2021) COVID-19 vaccination programme: development, distribution, data. https://ukhsa.blog.gov.uk/2021/12/08/14634/

UK Health Security Agency (2024). Chapter 15a Dengue. https://travelhealthpro.org.uk/media_lib/mlib-uploads/full/the-green-book-chapter-15a-dengue-october-2024.pdf

UK Health Security Agency (2025). Chapter 29. Smallpox and mpox. https://assets.publishing.service.gov.uk/media/67b4f1a44a80c6718b55bf5f/Green-Book-Chapter_29_Smallpox_and_mpox_18_February_2025.pdf

World Health Organization (2020). Ebola virus disease and vaccines Ebola virus disease: Vaccines

World Health Organization (2024a) History of Small pox vaccine on line https://www.who.int/news-room/spotlight/history-of-vaccination/history-of-smallpox-vaccination

World Health Organization (2024b) HIV and AIDS https://www.who.int/news-room/fact-sheets/detail/hiv-aids

World Health Organization (2024c) Disease outbreak Marburg virus disease - Rwanda https://www.who.int/emergencies/disease-outbreak-news/item/2024-DON544

World Health Organization (2024d) Statement of the fortieth meeting of the Polio IHR Emergency Committee Statement of the fortieth meeting of the Polio IHR Emergency Committee

World Health Organization (No date). Coronavirus Disease (COVID-19) Pandemic. https://www.who.int/europe/emergencies/situations/covid-19

Additional Reading

Pollard, A.J. and Bijker, E.M., 2021. A guide to vaccinology: from basic principles to new developments. *Nature Reviews Immunology*, *21*(2), pp.83-100.

References

NHS (2023) NHS Constitution for England https://www.gov.uk/government/publications/the-nhs-constitution-for-england (accessed 04/11/2024)

UKHSA (Online): The Green Book Immunisation against infectious disease https://www.gov.uk/government/collections/immunisation-against-infectious-disease-the-green-book (accessed 04/11/2024)

Vaccine Development and Onward Management of Vaccine Safety

3

Karen Ford and Rachel White

3.1 Introduction

Understanding how vaccines work, the different types of vaccines, their constituents and the reasons why we give them is essential part of the vaccination process. Nurses need to be familiar with this information so that they can answer any questions that may arise and be confident themselves of the safety and effectiveness of the vaccines they are administering. Being able to explain how vaccines are developed and the ongoing management of vaccine safety is an important part of the process in maintaining people's trust and confidence in vaccine programmes.

More detailed information can be found in the further resources section.

3.2 How Do Vaccines Work?

To understand vaccine safety, it is first important to understand how vaccines work. The process of vaccination mimics the body's own natural response to infections by stimulating the immune system.

The immune system identifies and destroys harmful foreign organisms (pathogens) that enter the body—these include the bacteria or viruses which cause vaccine preventable diseases.

The immune system's response is complex (see Fig. 3.1)—it can be summarised as follows:

- A bacteria or virus enters the body (antigen).

K. Ford (✉) · R. White (✉)
The Oxford Vaccine Group, University of Oxford, London, UK
e-mail: Karen.ford@paediatrics.ox.ac.uk; Rachel.white@paediatrics.ox.ac.uk

© Springer Nature Switzerland AG 2025
H. Donovan, H. Bedford (eds.), *Safe Vaccine Administration*,
https://doi.org/10.1007/978-3-031-92498-9_3

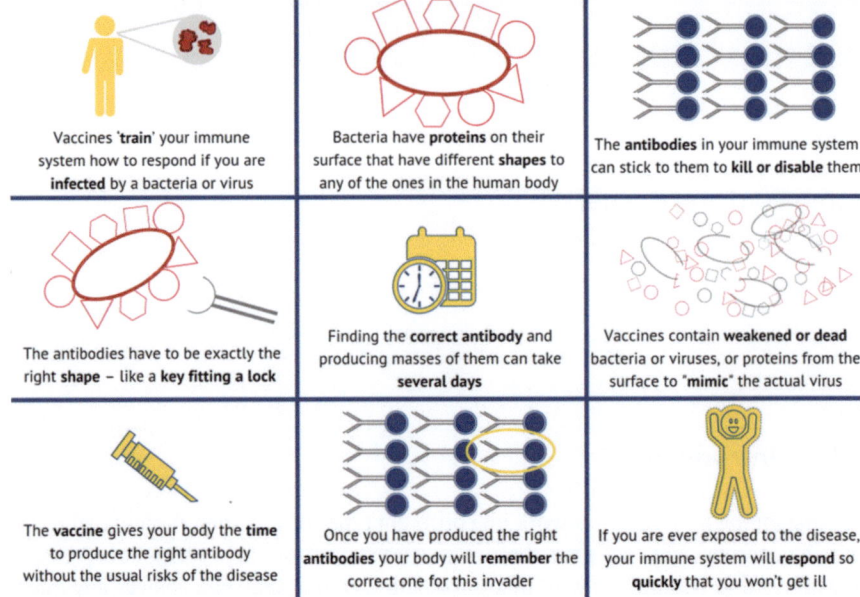

Fig. 3.1 How vaccines work (Diagram credited to "Vaccine Knowledge" courtesy of Tatjana Marks)

- Specialised cells of the immune system recognise bacterial or viral proteins (antigens) and stimulate other immune cells to produce antibodies (a type of protective protein).
- Lymphocytes (specialised white blood cells) identify and mark the antigen for destruction.
- Some of these lymphocytes develop into memory cells, known as T and B cells, which are able to remain in the body for very long periods of time and recognise these specific antigens in the future if the body encounters that pathogen again.
- Development of memory cells allows the immune system to respond faster and more effectively on second or subsequent encounters with these specific antigens.

The aim of a vaccine is to stimulate the immune system to develop long-lasting immunity against antigens from the specific bacteria or virus that causes disease without having to suffer the ill effects and risks of the natural infection.

A successful immune response to a vaccine antigen means that when the individual is exposed again to the antigen, either naturally or by a subsequent vaccine dose, a much stronger, faster and effective immune response will result as the immune system has been primed to combat the disease. The body's response to a vaccine mimics its natural reaction to infection. Vaccines train the immune system so that is it is ready to respond.

As vaccination aims to elicit an immune response, some adverse reactions (such as feeling tired or generally unwell, even getting a slight fever afterward) are expected, just as they would following natural infection. The vaccine development process carefully monitors these adverse reactions through clinical trials. Ongoing safety vigilance ensures that the risks of vaccine adverse reactions compared to the risks of natural infection achieve an acceptable balance.

3.3 What Is the Ideal Vaccine?

Manufacturers endeavour to achieve several characteristics in the development and production of vaccines (World Health Organization et al. 2013).

These include the following:

- Prevent or reduce severity of infectious disease.
- Provoke the immune system to provide durable and long-term protection to the disease.
- Minimal doses of vaccines required to provide immunity.
- Provide the broadest protection against disease.
- Cause minimal or no adverse reactions.
- Be stable at extremes of temperature over long periods of time to ease storage.
- Through mass production be available for widespread use.
- Be affordable.

To achieve these ambitions, several different types of vaccines exist reflecting the natural complexity of infectious disease.

3.4 What Are the Different Types of Vaccines?

Vaccines can be categorised into many types according to the biological features of the antigens and the technologies used during the preparation of the vaccines.

However, the two main defining groups are "live" (contain whole bacteria or viruses which have been weakened) and "non-live" (contain whole bacteria or viruses which have been killed through physical or chemical processes) (Oxford Vaccine Group 2021).

Pollard and Bijker (2020) provides an extensive overview of the different types of vaccines along with examples of licensed vaccines and is a highly recommended reading.

3.4.1 Combination Vaccines

Combination vaccines contain antigens to protect against two or more diseases, for example, the combined six in one vaccine which protects against diphtheria, tetanus, pertussis (whooping cough), polio, *Haemophilus influenzae* type b and hepatitis B (DTaP/IPV/Hib/HepB). Prior to licensing, manufacturers are required to extensively evaluate adverse reactions, the immune response evoked by each of the separate antigens within the combined vaccine and possible reactions between them. As with all vaccines, careful monitoring is required after licensing. It is not possible for all vaccines to be made into combinations. The benefits of combined vaccines include the following (World Health Organization et al. 2013):

- Reduced costs associated with storage, maintaining stock and administration compared to separate vaccines.
- Fewer visits to healthcare professionals are required and therefore potentially higher acceptance rates.
- More diseases can be protected against all at once allowing timely protection.
- The addition of new vaccines into the schedule may be facilitated by reducing the number of injections administered at one-time point while still protecting against the same number of infectious diseases.

> **Box 3.1 Summary Point**
> - The body's response to a vaccine mimics its natural reaction to infection.
> - There are many different types of vaccine; however, the two main distinctions are live and non-live.

3.5 What Do Vaccines Contain?

Below many vaccine ingredients are classified; however, the list is not exhaustive:

Vaccines contain one or more antigens and several added substances such as stabilizers, adjuvants and preservatives, which together are called excipients. There may also be residual components left over from the manufacturing processes such as small amounts of antibiotic.

The following link provides a guide of what a vaccine is made up of, including pictorial explanations: www.immunology.org/public-information/vaccine-resources/vaccines/vaccine-infographics/whats-vaccine.

All components of a vaccine are listed within the summary of product characteristics (SMPC). These can be accessed online on the electronic medicine's compendium: https://www.medicines.org.uk/emc. It is important for practitioners to know where to find information about vaccine components, as a severe hypersensitivity reaction to any of these can be a contraindication to receiving that particular vaccine.

Some important things to remember when considering vaccine ingredients are as follows:

- The main ingredient in vaccines is water. Most vaccines are a total volume of 0.5 mL (about the tip of a teaspoon) with a significant part of this being water for injection.

- Many of the other ingredients are found naturally within the body, such as sodium chloride, which is table salt and is an essential part of our bodies.
- The active ingredient is the part which induces the specific immune response. The amount of this is as small as possible and is established through research. Compared to the quantity of bacteria and viruses that our bodies are exposed to naturally within the environment, the amount of active ingredients found within vaccines is tiny.
- The quantity of added ingredients is very small often measured as nanograms ng (1 ng = 0.001 µg).
- Any manufacturing residuals will only be present as traces that are so small, they are difficult to measure.
- As vaccine research continues and our knowledge increases, we sometimes discover that the amount of active ingredient and other excipients can be reduced compared to what was used historically.

3.6 Added Ingredients

There are three main classifications of added ingredients: preservatives, adjuvants and stabilisers. Each has their own purpose as explained in Table 3.1.

In addition to these three main classifications, other ingredients can be added to some vaccines for a specific purpose, e.g. a taste enhancer is added to the oral rotavirus vaccine. As previously mentioned, vaccines may also contain traces of substances used within the manufacturing processes such as antibiotics (Table 3.1).

> A table summarising vaccine excipients within vaccines, by vaccine, used within the USA (many of which are also used within the UK) is published by the Centers for Disease Control and Prevention and may be useful for nurses in the UK as a reference: https://www.cdc.gov/vaccines/pubs/pinkbook/downloads/appendices/B/excipient-table-2.pdf

Table 3.1 Summary of the purposes of added ingredients and residual substances

Vaccine ingredient	Rationale for inclusion in vaccine and points to note	
Preservatives	Help to make the vaccine last longer "on the shelf" by preventing the growth of bacteria or fungi that may be unintentionally introduced into the vaccine during the manufacturing process (Dreher-Lesnick and Finn 2024)	
	Example **Thiomersal (thimerosal in the USA)** An ethyl mercury-containing compound Currently no vaccines within the UK routine immunisation schedule contain thiomersal, but it is widely used in many countries outside Europe and the USA	There has been considerable controversy around the use of thiomersal in vaccines. There was concern that it may be linked to autism and other neurodevelopmental disorders in children (Dreher-Lesnick and Finn 2024). However, there is no evidence that this is the case (Taylor et al. 2014)
Adjuvants	Substances that enhance, accelerate or direct the immune response. These work in tandem with the antigen	
	Example **Aluminium salts: aluminium hydroxide, aluminium phosphate and potassium aluminium sulphate** Aluminium is an element which is released naturally into the environment via volcanic activity and the breaking down of rocks Aluminium salts slow down the escape of the vaccine antigen from the site of injection; this increases the length of contact between the antigen and the immune system such as macrophages and other antigen-receptive cells (World Health Organization et al. 2013)	There has been public concerns surrounding aluminium in vaccines, wrongly linked to autism and neurological issues. However, in June 2012 the Global Advisory Committee on Vaccine Safety (GACVS) concluded that the data they reviewed did not raise concerns about the safety of aluminium in vaccines: https://www.who.int/groups/global-advisory-committee-on-vaccine-safety/committee-reports

(continued)

Table 3.1 (continued)

Stabilisers	Help maintain the vaccine's effectiveness during storage. Temperature, acidity or alkalinity all affect vaccine stability (World Health Organization et al. 2013). Types of substances used in vaccines as stabilisers include sugars and proteins	
	Example **Gelatine** Gelatine originates from the collagen, found within the tendons, ligaments, bones and cartilage of animals Porcine gelatine used in some vaccines is derived from pigs, manufactured under strict hygiene and safety regulations, highly purified and hydrolysed (broken down by water) into very small molecules called peptides (UK Health Security Agency, 2022b)	The acceptance of vaccines that contain gelatine may be of concern to members of some religious communities or cultural groups. UK Health Security Agency has produced a leaflet to address this issue (available in several languages): https://www.gov.uk/government/publications/vaccines-and-porcine-gelatine
Manufacturing residuals	Products used in the manufacturing processes of vaccines may remain as trace elements within the final vaccine and are referred to as residuals Various steps in the manufacturing process will aim to remove or reduce the amount of residual; however, it is not always possible to remove them completely nor demonstrate definitively that it has been completely removed (Dreher-Lesnick and Finn 2024) The purposes of these potential residual products include inactivation of a virus, prevention of bacterial contamination, medium for growing cell lines and viruses	
Purpose: inactivation of virus or detoxifying toxin	**Examples: inactivation residual** **Formaldehyde** This is a naturally occurring compound present in the human body as the result of various biochemical processes (Heck et al. 1990): • In vaccines, it is used to: inactivate viruses (e.g. inactivated polio vaccine) • Make toxins less harmful such as diphtheria and tetanus toxins	Most formaldehyde is removed from vaccines by purification processes during production—that which remains is several hundred times lower than the amount known to do harm to humans (World Health Organization et al. 2013)

(continued)

Table 3.1 (continued)

Purpose: prevention of bacterial growth	**Example** **Antibiotics** Used to prevent bacterial contamination of the culture cells in which the viruses to be used within vaccines are grown (World Health Organization et al. 2013). Antibiotics that have been used for this purpose include streptomycin, polymyxin B, neomycin and gentamicin (Dreher-Lesnick and Finn 2024)	Antibiotics associated with common allergic reactions are avoided, for example, the Code of Federal Regulations—USA—does not permit the use of penicillin in vaccines (Dreher-Lesnick and Finn 2024)
Medium for growth of cell line	**Example** **Yeast** The immunogenic antigen of some vaccines is produced in yeast cells (*Saccharomyces cerevisiae*) using recombinant DNA technology	Some brands of inactivated influenza vaccines use cell lines to produce the influenza virus used within the vaccine
Medium for growing virus	**Example: egg protein (ovalbumin)** The influenza viruses contained within numerous influenza vaccines are grown on fertilised hen's egg. As result, there may be ovalbumin (egg proteins) contained with the vaccines	The management of individuals with egg allergy who require influenza vaccination is outlined within the influenza chapter of *Immunisation Against Infectious Diseases*: www.gov.uk/government/publications/influenza-the-green-book-chapter-19 Influenza vaccines produced using cell line technologies are egg-free Seasonal influenza immunisation details are published here at www.gov.uk/government/collections/immunisation

3.7 How Are Vaccines Tested and Trialled?

For a vaccine to be used in the UK, it must have a licence or marketing authorisation. The Medicines and Health Care Products Regulatory Agency (MHRA), a government body, regulates and monitors the marketing authorisation process in the UK. Prior to a vaccine being licenced, they are thoroughly trialled on thousands of people and must meet rigorous safety standards. It is not possible to produce a vaccine completely free of risk. However, the MHRA are responsible for ensuring that these risks are minimised by using sound evidence to underpin and support decisions that the organisation makes (MRHA, 2023).

A vaccine is only granted a licence after it has met a high standard of safety and quality and is thought to be effective for its intended purpose in the intended population. In order to achieve this, there are several clinical trial phases that must be carried out: preclinical, phase I, phase II, phase III and phase IV—these will be explained later in this chapter.

The requirements of a large and detailed regulatory framework must be met during trial development and for the duration of the trial. Evidence showing that a trial team is constantly meeting these requirements must be provided and is part of the application process to the MHRA.

The term "sponsor" is used to refer to the *company, institution or organisation which takes responsibility for the initiation, management and/or financing of a clinical trial*. For a vaccine trial to be conducted in humans, the first stage is for the sponsor, e.g. pharmaceutical company or research institution, to apply to the MHRA for permission to conduct the trial in the UK.

Examples of the extensive regulation and where to find further information can be found in Table 3.2.

Table 3.2 Summary of regulation and governance for medical research and further reading

Regulation and governance	
International Council of Harmonisation Good Clinical Practice (ICH GCP)	Ethical and scientific quality standard for the conduct of trials human participants (European Medicines Agency 2025 https://www.ema.europa.eu/en/documents/scientific-guideline/ich-e-6-r2-guideline-good-clinical-practice-step-5_en.pdf)
Declaration of Helsinki	Ethical principles for medical research involving human participants (ref https://www.wma.net/what-we-do/medical-ethics/declaration-of-helsinki/)
Medicines for Human Use (Clinical Trials) Regulations 2004	http://www.legislation.gov.uk/uksi/2004/1031/contents/made
European Union trials direction	Incorporated into UK law by the Medicine for Human Use (Clinical Trials) Regulations (THE EUROPEAN PARLIAMENT AND THE COUNCIL OF THE EUROPEAN UNION 16th April 2014, https://ec.europa.eu/health/sites/health/files/files/eudralex/vol-1/reg_2014_536/reg_2014_536_en.pdf
Royal College of Paediatrics and Child Health guidelines for the ethical conduct of medical research involving children 2000	https://adc.bmj.com/content/archdischild/82/2/177.full.pdf
Databases and further reading	
Clinical Trials.gov	A registry and results database of publicly and privately supported clinical trials of human participants conducted around the world
ISRCTN	A clinical trial registry recognised by WHO and ICMJE (a small group of general medical journal editors and representatives of selected related organisations) that accepts all clinical research studies (whether proposed, ongoing or completed), providing content validation and curation and the unique identification number necessary for publication
EudraCT	European Clinical Trials Database of all clinical trials of investigational medicinal products, with at least one site in the European Union commencing May 1, 2004, or later

In addition, the trial plan must be presented to a National Health Service (NHS) Health Research Authority ethics committee, as well as a local NHS Research and Development office, and for some trials, Health and Safety Executive (HSE) review. All these bodies must give their approval for a trial to commence.

For some clinical trials of vaccines, before issuing approval for the trial, the MHRA will seek expert advice from the Clinical Trials, Biologicals and Vaccines Expert Advisory Group (CTBVEAG) of the Commission on Human Medicines (CHM). The MHRA make their decision to seek expert advice based on an assessment of the risks involved within the trial and how the sponsor of the trial plans to mitigate them.

The many stages of regulation governing the conduct of clinical trials are portrayed within the National Institute of Health Research (NIHR) clinical trials toolkit route map: http://www.ct-toolkit.ac.uk/routemap/.

The underpinning paradigm of the regulations involving the conduct of clinical vaccine trials is to ensure the safety of the trial participants and ensure that the knowledge output of the trial will be of a high, reliable standard on which clinical decisions and guidance can be made. The heart of all the regulations, guidance and legislation which govern the conduct of any clinical research are the Principles of International Council of Harmonisation Good Clinical Practice (ICH-GCP) (European Medicines Agency 2023). There are 13 core principles of ICH-GCP. Two of the most important core principles of GCP are as follows:

- The rights, safety and well-being of the trial participants are the most important considerations and should prevail over the interests of science and society.
- Freely given informed consent should be obtained from every subject prior to clinical trial participation.

The MHRA gives overarching approval for a clinical trial to be conducted. Clinical trials of vaccines must be registered on a widely accessible database to aid in the transparency of research and the results it generates aiding the creation of an unbiased and complete evidence base. See example databases in Table 3.2.

3.8 Phases of Clinical Trials

Several clinical trial phases take place prior to licensure of a vaccine, the first being known as preclinical. Prior to a vaccine being given to humans, the immunogenic (able to produce an immune response) antigen will have been trialled in animals to provide an indication of safety and to ensure that it provokes an immune response.

The Veterinary Medicines Directorate, a government body, regulates and oversees these trials (Gov.uk. Veterinary Medicines Directorate 2020).

Following on from this phase of preclinical work, vaccine trials may then be conducted in humans (phase I–IV), with each phase progressively increasing the number of participants they include.

The vaccine being developed or progressed within a clinical trial is referred to as the investigational medicinal product (IMP).

The clinical trial design used to test vaccines is often a randomised controlled trial (RCT). Participants are randomly allocated to receive either the vaccine being developed (or the new vaccine schedule being developed) or to a "control"—this control can be to receive a vaccine that is already licensed or may be a placebo (a substance that has no action), such as sterile water. The group to which participants are assigned are often referred to as the "arms" of a trial.

Hackshaw (2011) provides an overview of the different stages of clinical trials (summarised in Table 3.3).

It can generally take several decades to develop and trial a vaccine before it is granted a licence. There are several related factors which made it possible to develop vaccines to protect against COVID-19 in a much shorter timeframe:

Table 3.3 Summary of the phases of clinical trials

Phase	Explanation
Phase I ↓	• First in humans • Very few participants • Assess vaccine safety and effectiveness (biological and pharmacological effects) • Evidence of provoking immune response needs to be seen • Generally trialled in young, healthy adults with close monitoring of participants for safety and general health of participants
Phase II ↓	• Larger participant numbers • Establishment that vaccine works and preliminary efficacy results • Identify common short-term side effects • Generate more safety data • Participants tend to be the age group for which the vaccine is eventually intended • Different groups within the trial to establish different formulas/compare a previous unvaccinated group
Phase III ↓	• Several hundred to thousands of participants in order to generate reliable data • Recruitment often over more than one site/country • Can take several years for completion • Other routine vaccines are also provided within trial, at same time as the IMP if applicable to ensure no undesired interaction between vaccines • Provides further data on how well the vaccine works (immunogenicity) • Provides more detailed safety data, e.g. expected longevity of side effects • Provides more data on local side effects and likelihood of temperature postvaccination (reactogenicity data) • Data from phase III trials inform the labelling, SmPC and patient leaflet information once vaccine is licensed • Licensing tends to occur once phase III trials are completed

(continued)

Table 3.3 (continued)

Phase	Explanation
Licence and vaccine in use	• After completion of phase III, the vaccine is reviewed for licensing and use
Phase IV (300 plus)	• Referred to as post-marketing or surveillance studies • Very large sample size (several hundred/thousand) • Often use multiple sites to recruit • Primary aim—continue monitoring efficacy and safety post licensure of vaccine • Answer new scientific questions to inform vaccination policy

- The vaccines were based on technologies that had been investigated over many preceding years.
- Priority was given to research relating to COVID-19 by all organisations and authorities involved in the research process.
- The above meant that other research trials were paused and more staff were available to assist in working on COVID-19 trials.
- Any changes to the trial (i.e. when new data surfaced) resulted in a trial paused for 6 weeks and regulatory bodies prioritised the review.
- Due to the high media profile, volunteers came forward quickly to participate in the COVID-19 vaccine trials enabling rapid recruitment of participant numbers to these trials.

After licensing the vaccine is used more generally by a wider population group; this can identify additional side effects that were not identified by the research trials due to the practical limits on the number of participants that can be included within the trial. The MHRA also oversees the safety of vaccines once licensed via the yellow card reporting system (see later).

One of the key elements of these clinical trials at each phase is that they are all guided by a carefully written protocol. This protocol states how a clinical trial will be undertaken and will determine if it is feasible in practice (the core document reviewed by the regulatory bodies).

There are four key design features that inform the protocol according to Hackshaw (2011): inclusion and exclusion criteria, control group, randomisation and blinding (Table 3.4).

3 Vaccine Development and Onward Management of Vaccine Safety   71

Table 3.4 Key design features that inform clinical trial protocols

Four key design features			
Inclusion and exclusion criteria	Control group	Randomisation	Blinding

• A criterion set that must be fulfilled in order for an individual to be eligible to participate
• Clinical trial phase and trial objectives determine the inclusion and exclusion criteria, e.g. age range, no underlying medical conditions, available for all study visits, no contraindications to IMP/routine vaccines provided
• Consideration of advantages and disadvantages required regarding the group selected, e.g.
  – Phase I—very strict eligibility due to first in humans, requiring very healthy participants who have undergone safety screening prior to full enrolment
  – Phase III and IV inclusion and exclusion criteria less restrictive, resulting in a more representative sample of participants from a wider population
	• Arm of a study where the participants do not receive the new intervention, instead receive either the current standard of care, no intervention or a placebo
	• This allows for comparison of outcomes between those that received the IMP and those that did not
	• Vaccine trials often favour giving a licensed vaccine within the control (rather than placebo) to provide some benefit to the participant undergoing the process of injection
		• Allocation of participants to different arms, which have different interventions
		• Aim is to produce groups of participants similar in terms of characteristics
		• It minimises bias
		This allows any differences in outcomes of the trial to be attributed to the intervention and not differences in the characteristics of the participants within different arms
			• Concealing the intervention received by participant
			• Double blinded – neither participant nor researchers involved in administrating the vaccine, managing or assessing the participant have knowledge of the intervention received by the participant
			• Single blinded – only the participant is unaware of what intervention they have received
			• Blinding aids the reduction of bias, e.g. the placebo effect, referring to the psychological ability to affects one's own health status

Box 3.2 Summary Points Regarding Clinical Trials
- Clinical trials are heavily regulated to ensure participant safety and the creation of reliable data to evaluate new vaccines, new vaccine schedules and unanswered scientific questions.
- The number of participants within a clinical trial increases with the phase of the trial.
- The design of a vaccine trial is often a randomised controlled trial as this design generates strong evidence.

3.9 Assessing Immunogenicity of a Vaccine Within Clinical Trials

Immunogenicity refers to the ability of a vaccine to provoke an immune response in the person immunised. The immune response will be directed toward the antigen(s) present in the vaccine. Within clinical trials, immunogenicity is measured in different ways. The primary method involves collecting blood from participants before vaccination and at several time points afterward. The blood is then analysed for different markers of immune responses, for example, antibodies and different types of cells, such as T and B cells which are important parts of the immune responses.

Instead of measuring the immune response, one can also measure the efficacy of a vaccine. This is how well the vaccine actually prevents the target disease. This can be measured in different ways:

- Prevention of a marker of disease, for example, during the development of the human papilloma virus vaccine, waiting to measure cases of cervical cancer would not have been ethical, so the vaccine was evaluated based on its ability to prevent precancerous lesions instead (UKHSA 2023).

3.10 Collecting Safety Data Within Clinical Trials

3.10.1 How Are Adverse Events After Vaccination Assessed?

An adverse event following immunisation (AEFI) is a term used to describe any untoward medical occurrence which follows a person being immunised, but was not necessarily caused by the vaccine. The adverse event may be any unfavourable or unintended sign, abnormal laboratory finding, symptom or disease (World Health Organization 2016).

The World Health Organization (2016) gives five categories of AEFI (Table 3.5) (management of these is discussed in Chap. 10 of this book):
Other things to note

- It is common for injectable vaccines to cause some adverse events such as redness, swelling and tenderness around an injection site (UK Health Security Agency, 2019).
- The aim is to ensure that the resulting adverse vaccine reactions occur at a frequency and severity that is considered acceptable when one weighs these against the benefits of vaccination while always producing the best possible immune response.

Table 3.5 AEFI categories

Category	AEFI caused or precipitated by
Vaccine product-related reaction	A vaccine due to one or more of the inherent properties of the vaccine. Example: redness around an injection site
Vaccine quality defect-related reaction	A vaccine that due to one or more quality defects of the vaccine product including its administration device as provided by the manufacturer
Immunisation error-related reaction	Inappropriate vaccine handling, prescribing or administration which could have been avoided. Example: administration of compromised vaccine due to unnoticed break in the cold chain
Immunisation anxiety-related reaction	Anxiety about the immunisation. Example: vasovagal syncope in an adolescent during or straight after vaccination
Coincidental event	Something other than the vaccine product, immunisation error or immunisation anxiety. Example: a fever that occurs on the day of vaccine (temporal association) but is caused by a recently caught viral illness

Table 3.6 Summary for capturing adverse events during clinical trials

Method	Examples of data captured
Participant diary records	Potential anticipated reactions such as local vaccine site reactions, e.g. redness, swelling and tenderness and systemic reactions such as temperature, malaise, tiredness, headache, loss of appetite. In addition, any other adverse events are captured and medication used to treat them, for example, chest infection and antibiotic use
Regular participant review to indicate safety measures	Generally, face-to-face appointments but sometimes phone calls—all recorded on databases. This allows for assessment of • General health • Baseline bloods for initial eligibility assessment • Follow-up bloods throughout the trial period to detect clinically significant changes • Review of adverse events and serious adverse events (see below)

3.10.2 How Are Adverse Events Captured in Clinical Trials?

During clinical trials, adverse reactions are captured in many ways as outlined in Table 3.6.

3.10.3 Serious Adverse Events (SAEs)

An SAE is an untoward medical occurrence with any dose (MHRA, 2021b, pg. 138):

- Results in death
- Is life-threatening
- Requires inpatient hospitalisation or prolongation of existing hospitalisation

- Results in persistent or significant disability or incapacity
- Consists of a congenital anomaly or birth defect

At all visits and points of contact during a clinical vaccine trial, participants are asked by research staff whether any SAEs have occurred and the details. These data are always collected, even if it is evident that there is no connection with the trial vaccine (IMP).

Other related SAE points

- All SAEs reported within a trial will be reviewed by the data safety committee (a separate group of experts from the trial (Wilhelmsen, 2002)) responsible for the trial.
- In later stage trials (phase III/IV), expected occurrences of events that would be considered serious but are known to occur within the eligible trial population may be exempt from being reported as an SAE; these events will be predefined within the clinical trial protocol.
- Often participants will be followed up by research staff for a year or longer after all vaccine doses. If no face-to-face contact is required (e.g. to collect study samples such as blood), a safety phone call may be sufficient.
- Even within phase IV vaccine trials, using licensed vaccine, SAEs will be captured, whereas expected adverse vaccine reactions may not be. By capturing all SAEs within these phase IV trials, additional safety data is captured post licensing.

3.10.4 SAE Reporting

There is strict regulation regarding the prompt reporting of SAEs by the research study centre to the sponsor of the clinical trial. Once the study site becomes aware of an SAE, the following takes place:

- An initial report is submitted to the sponsor within 24 h.
- The principal investigator of the clinical trials takes overall responsibility or delegates this responsibility to appropriately trained staff, who assess the seriousness of the adverse event and if it is, or is not, related to the IMP.
- If an SAE is considered related to the IMP and is not an expected reaction, it is defined as an SUSAR—a Suspected Unexpected Serious Adverse Event.
- The MHRA and ethics committee must be notified of all SUSARs.
- For SUSARs that are fatal or life-threatening, reporting must happen within 7 days—all other SUSARs need to be reported within 15 days.
- In extenuating circumstances, a SUSAR may result in the temporary halt, early termination or the trial not recommencing.

Information gathered through the reporting of SAEs and SUSARs is reported in annual safety reports in the form of a Development Safety Update Report (DSUR).

The number of participants who have received the trial vaccine (IMP) is included within this report. The aim of a DSUR is to describe concisely all new safety information relevant to the IMP. The DSUR is submitted to the MHRA and the ethics committee.

3.11 How Is the Decision to Grant a Licence for a Vaccine Taken?

A licence or marketing authorisation for new vaccines is awarded by the MHRA or the European regulator—EMA (Fig. 3.2).

Experts from different relevant specialties who have undergone additional training in medicines assessment make up the assessment team. The role of the assessment teams is to ensure the following:

- Trial data shows that the vaccine meets acceptable levels of safety, immunogenicity or efficacy.
- For most people, the advantages of the vaccine far outweigh any disadvantages.

Once the MHRA and EMA are convinced that these criteria have been met, it will issue a licence provided they are satisfied that the manufacture, distribution and supply of the vaccine will meet the required safety and quality standards (Medicines and Healthcare products Regulatory Agency, 2014).

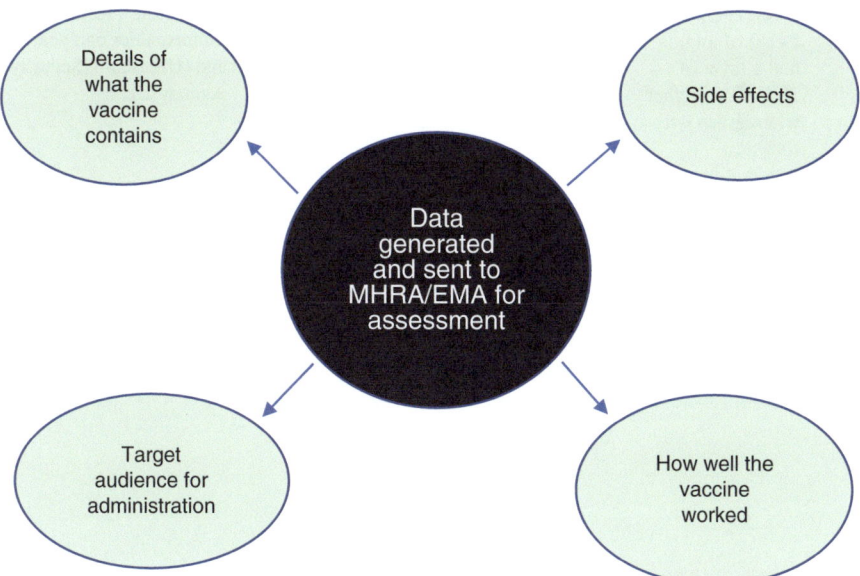

Fig. 3.2 Process for licence or market authorisation

3.12 Why Is It Important to Know the Possible Expected Adverse Events Following Vaccination?

Knowing what possible expected adverse events may occur after vaccination can inform the advice health professionals give to parents/carers. People who then receive the vaccine know what kind of side effects to expect postvaccination. Being informed of possible adverse events can help to reduce anxiety if they do occur and confer public confidence in vaccines. For example, the frequency of injection site reactions following an adjuvant inactivated influenza vaccine is more common than after a non-adjuvant inactivated influenza vaccine (UK Health Security Agency, 2022a).

Additionally, safety data from vaccine research trials can influence vaccine policy as illustrated by the examples (Tables 3.7 and 3.8):

Table 3.7 4CMen B (Bexsero®) and prophylactic paracetamol

Findings	Concerns	Further trials	Outcome
A clinically relevant systemic reaction of high fevers following infant immunisation with 4CMen B vaccine (when given alongside routine vaccinations) was discovered (Gossger et al. 2012); • 77% (1912 of 2478) of infants had a fever of 38.5 °C or higher when given with routine vaccinations • 45% (295 of 659) after routine vaccines alone This meant that around three quarters of all infants immunised had a significant fever (Vesikari et al. 2013)	Not having been perceived as an acceptable side effect of vaccination by parents or health professionals	Further clinical trials carried out demonstrated that prophylactic paracetamol administration reduced the frequency of high temperatures without affecting the immunogenicity of 4CMen B and other routine infant vaccines, when administered concomitantly (Prymula et al. 2014)	With the introduction of 4CMen B vaccine into the UK immunisation schedule in 2015 routine practice change to recommending prophylactic paracetamol when 4CMenB is given with the routine vaccines in infants under one year of age (UK Health Security Agency 2022b)

Table 3.8 Upper age limit for administration of rotavirus due to risk of intussusception

Findings	Outcome
Data from observational safety studies carried out in several countries indicated a small increased risk of intussusception occurring, mainly within seven days after vaccination with Rotarix® Up to 6 additional cases per 100,000 infants against a background incidence of 25 to 101 per 100,000 infants aged less than one per year (*Rotarix oral suspension in squeezable tube—Summary of Product Characteristics (SmPC)—(emc)*, no date) Occurrence of intussusception peaks at around 5 months in the UK (Ramsay and Waight 1999) • Rotavirus vaccination is contraindicated in infants with previous history or have a malformation of gastrointestinal tract (UK Health Security Agency 2015)	• The first dose of rotavirus vaccine Rotarix® should not be given after 15 weeks of age in the UK (UK Health Security Agency 2015) Not administering the first dose of rotavirus after 15 weeks of age reflects the possible risk of intussusception occurring which is more likely to occur naturally as the infant gets older; in addition, it helps to reduce the possibility of a temporal association of intussusception with the vaccine

> **Box 3.3 Key Summary Points for Clinical Trial Governance and Reporting**
> - There are comprehensive requirements and legislation governing the capture and reporting of safety data within clinical vaccine trials.
> - Adverse event data gathered in clinical trials inform advice given, regarding potential vaccine side effects as well as vaccine policy.
> - All data gathered through clinical trials are reviewed by expert teams within the Medicines and HealthCare production Regulatory Agency (MHRA) or European Medicines Agency (EMA) prior to a vaccine being licensed or given marketing authorisation.

3.13 How Is the Safety of Vaccines Monitored Once Licensed?

Several steps and processes postvaccine licensure enable continued monitoring of safety. Safety information is gathered from a variety of sources including the yellow card scheme, medical literature, post-marketing safety studies, epidemiological databases and other worldwide organisations such as the Global Advisory Committee on Vaccine Safety (GACVS).

These processes are outlined in Table 3.9, along with links for further reading.

Table 3.9 Summary for postvaccine licence safety monitoring

Component	Explanation
Control testing of vaccine batches	The role of the National Institute for Biological Standards and Control (NIBSC) is the characterisation, standardisation and control of biological medicines (Medicines and Healthcare products Regulatory Agency undated)
Global Advisory Committee on Vaccine Safety (GACVS)	Established by the World Health Organization (WHO) in 1999. The committee advises the WHO on vaccine related safety issues, enabling it to respond promptly, efficiently and with scientific rigour to any safety issues that potentially could have global importance In the UK, the MHRA is responsible for monitoring the safety of all medicines including vaccines
The yellow card scheme	A voluntary reporting scheme of adverse drug reactions (ADRs), including AEFI, that are suspected to be vaccine induced When a vaccine is newly licensed, they are subject to enhanced surveillance and given "black triangle status" meaning all serious and non-serious suspected ADRs should be reported. Once a vaccine is no longer classified as "black triangle status", it is only serious ADRs that are expected to be reported https://yellowcard.mhra.gov.uk/
General Practice Research Database (GPRD)	Set up in 1987 and run by the MHRA, it is a database of anonymised data from a sample of patient records, collected from over 480 GPs in the UK The database is used for gathering information such as the following: • Investigating and monitoring side effects of medicines and vaccines • Causes of diseases • Associated risk factors
EudraVigilance	Analyses reports on adverse drug reactions

3.14 How Are Defects in a Vaccine or Batch Reported?

Potential defects to vaccines include particulate contamination or errors in the packing and labelling. Such errors are reported by healthcare professionals, when noticed, to the Defective Medicines Report Centre (DMRC) of the Medicines and Healthcare Products Regulatory Agency (MHRA 2021a, b).

3.15 How Are Defects in the Devices Used to Administer Vaccines Reported?

Needles, syringes, vials and ampoules are examples of devices used in immunisation programmes. Any faults or inconsistencies in these devices are reported to the medical devices Adverse Incident Centre (AIC) at the MHRA.

The MHRA review reports received to the DMRC and the AIC, and corrective action is taken when required. Detecting trends and highlighting inadequate manufacturing or supply systems which need resolving add to the network of schemes to ensure vaccine safety (UK Health Security Agency, 2013).

3.16 How Is a Potential Concern over Vaccine Safety Responded to?

When available evidence supports a causal association between a vaccine and reported adverse drug reactions, the Commission for Human Medicines (CHM) and JCVI may recommend actions to be taken. Evidence is reviewed from all credible sources, and consideration is given to balancing the benefits of vaccination versus risk (Gov.uk).

Based on the recommendations from the CHM and JCVI, regulatory actions may be taken by the MHRA which could involve withdrawal of the vaccine or an amendment to the vaccine licence to ensure that it is used as safely and effectively as possible. If further evidence eliminates a causal association between a vaccine and an adverse drug reaction, previous restrictive actions could be removed.

As described in this chapter, the UK has comparable procedures to those in US governing processes for the continual monitoring of vaccine safety.

An example of this can be seen in Table 3.10, which outlines a timeline of a reactive safety review of the yellow fever vaccine (Stamaril®). The yellow fever vaccine is a vaccine administered on a selective programme, based on risk assessment related to travel outside the UK (UK Health Security Agency, 2020).

Table 3.10 Case study—timeline of ongoing review of vaccine safety of yellow fever vaccine

Date	Review	Outcome
2001	Review of evidence by the UK Committee on Safety of Medicines (CSM) and its Sub-Committee on Pharmacovigilance (SCOP)	Summary of Product Characteristics (SmPC) changed to include warnings of a precaution about use in subjects aged 60 years and older
2005	Review by Committee on Safety of Medicines (CSM) case reports vaccine-associated viscerotropic adverse reactions (YEL-AVD), had a history of thymus disorder	SmPC changed to include thymus dysfunction as a contraindication; warnings on the risks were expanded
2005	European article 30 referral to the European Medicines Agency (EMA). This type of referral is triggered when member states have adopted different decisions, e.g. different contraindications, and there is a need for them to be harmonised	SmPC harmonised across the European Union including recommendation that the vaccine should only be given to the elderly (from 60 years of age) if particular risk
September 3, 2007	Date of first authorisation/renewal of the authorisation of Stamaril®	

(continued)

Table 3.10 (continued)

Date	Review	Outcome
2013	WHO Strategic Advisory Group of Experts on Immunisation (SAGE) Working Group on yellow fever vaccines updated their recommendations	Vaccine offers a life-long protection against yellow fever. A booster dose is not generally needed, except for risk groups (60 years and above) based on a careful risk-benefit assessment
2013–2018	Through yellow card reporting to MHRA, the total of suspected adverse drug reactions for yellow fever vaccine was less than 40 per year following administration of approximately 140,000 doses per year	
2018–2019	Two fatal reports of yellow fever vaccine-associated neurotropic disease in the UK. Analysis by the official medicines control laboratory of samples from the batches implicated in the two fatal cases did not reveal unusual findings	
2019	MHRA convene expert group to review risk-benefit and risk minimisation for vaccine. Meet May, July and October	
January 3, 2019	Online Green Book Chap. 35, Yellow Fever, Stamaril® vaccine contraindication section updated for thymectomy and incidental thymectomy	
February 6, 2019	Joint Committee on Vaccination and Immunisation meeting report from MHRA, consulting JCVI on safety on vaccine	
April 16, 2019	Drug safety update from MHRA for Stamaril®	Vaccine contraindicated in individuals with medical history of thymus dysfunction or who are immunosuppressed
November 2019	Yellow fever vaccine—report of the Commission on Human Medicines Expert Working Group on Benefit-Risk and Risk Minimisation Measures Published	Key recommendations updated, such as contraindications and strengthened precautions
November 21, 2019	Drug safety update from MHRA for Stamaril®	Mirrors recommendations within CHM report issued November 2019
November 21, 2019	Online Green Book Chap. 35, Yellow Fever, updated to add guidance for Stamaril® for those with weakened immune systems, those over 60 years and anyone who has had their thymus removed	
Further reading	• Yellow-Fever-Vaccine-EWG-report__002_.pdf (publishing.service.gov.uk) • https://www.gov.uk/drug-safety-update/yellow-fever-vaccine-stamaril-and-fatal-adverse-reactions-extreme-caution-needed-in-people-who-may-be-immunosuppressed-and-those-60-years-and-older • https://www.gov.uk/government/groups/joint-committee-on-vaccination-and-immunisation • https://www.gov.uk/government/publications/yellow-fever-the-green-book-chapter-35 • https://www.gov.uk/government/publications/report-of-the-commission-on-human-medicines-expert-working-group-on-benefit-risk-and-risk-minimisation-measures-of-the-yellow-fever-vaccine	

Key Message
Wild-type yellow fever infection is a serious infection with a high mortality. The evidence on the ability of yellow fever vaccines to protect individuals vaccinated is robust; however, there are very rare life-threatening adverse drug reactions. Due to this, contraindications and precautions to receiving yellow fever vaccine must be followed. Like all vaccines, safety of yellow fever vaccines is being continually monitored.

Box 3.4 Summary of Key Points for Ongoing Safety Monitoring
- Multiple schemes monitor the safety of vaccines and gather evidence of potential issues. These include yellow card reporting system, General Practice Research Database, Case reports within Medical Literature, Eudra Vigilance, Defective Medicines Report Centre and Medical Devices Adverse Incident Centre
- Multiple establishments and organisations are involved in reviewing the evidence of vaccine safety including the Medicines and Healthcare Products Regulatory Agency (MHRA), Commission for Human Medicines (CHM) Gov.UK, Joint Committee on Vaccination and Immunisation (JCVI), European Medicines Agency (EMA) and the World Health Organization Global Advisory Committee on Vaccine Safety (GACVS)

Patients and parents should be reassured that there is a network of credible and auditable regulatory schemes that continually monitor the safety of vaccines after they have been licensed.

References

Dreher-Lesnick SM., and Finn TM. (Eds Orenstein WA., Offit PA., Edwards KM., Plotkin SA.) Vaccine additives and Manufacturing residuals in vaccines licensed in the United States. In Vaccines (Chapter 8) 2024. Elsevier 8th Edition

European Medicines Agency (2023) Good clinical practice -. https://www.ema.europa.eu/en/human-regulatory/research-development/compliance/good-clinical-practice (accessed 22/6/24)

European Medicines Agency (EMA). (2025). ICH E6 good clinical practice - Scientific guideline | European Medicines Agency (EMA). [online] Available at: https://www.ema.europa.eu/en/ich-e6-good-clinical-practicescientific-guideline

Gossger, N. *et al.* (2012) "Immunogenicity and tolerability of recombinant serogroup B meningococcal vaccine administered with or without routine infant vaccinations according to different immunization schedules," *JAMA*, 307(6). https://doi.org/10.1001/jama.2012.85

Gov.UK. The commission on Human Medicines. https://www.gov.uk/government/organisations/commission-on-human-medicines/about. (accessed 21/6/24)

Gov.uk. Veterinary Medicines Directorate (2020) Veterinary Medicines Directorate annual report and accounts 2019 to 2020 https://www.gov.uk/government/publications/veterinary-medicines-directorate-annual-report-and-accounts-2019-to-2020 (accessed 212/6/24)

Hackshaw, A. (2011) *A concise guide to clinical trials*. John Wiley & Sons.

Heck, H.D., Casanova, M. and Starr, T.B. (1990) "Formaldehyde Toxicity—New Understanding," *Critical Reviews in Toxicology*, 20(6), pp. 397–426. https://doi.org/10.3109/10408449009029329

Medicines and Healthcare Products Regulatory Agency (2021a). *Good clinical practice guide.* 12th edition. London: Medicines And Healthcare Products Regulatory Agency.

Medicines and Healthcare products Regulatory Agency (2021b) "A guide to defective medicinal products," *GOV.UK* Available at: https://www.gov.uk/government/publications/a-guide-to-defective-medicinal-products

MRHA 2023. More information about the MRHA https://www.gov.uk/government/publications/more-information-about-the-mhra/more-information-about-the-mhra%2D%2D2 accessed 21/6/24

Medicines and Healthcare products Regulatory Agency (undated) NIBSC - About us https://www.nibsc.org/about_us.aspx (accessed 21/6/24)

Oxford Vaccine Group (2021). Vaccine Knowledge. Types of vaccine. https://vaccineknowledge.ox.ac.uk/types-of-vaccine (accessed 22/6/24)

Pollard, A.J. and Bijker, E.M. (2020) "A guide to vaccinology: from basic principles to new developments," *Nature Reviews Immunology*, 21(2), pp. 83–100. https://doi.org/10.1038/s41577-020-00479-7

Prymula, R. *et al.* (2014) "A phase 2 randomized controlled trial of a multicomponent meningococcal serogroup B vaccine (I)," *Human Vaccines & Immunotherapeutics*, 10(7), pp. 1993–2004. Available at: https://doi.org/10.4161/hv.28666

Ramsay, M. and Waight, P. (1999) "Rotavirus vaccination and intussusception," *The Lancet*, 354(9182), p. 956. https://doi.org/10.1016/s0140-6736(05)75710-x

Taylor, L., Swerdfeger, A.L. and Eslick, G.D. (2014) "Vaccines are not associated with autism: An evidence-based meta-analysis of case-control and cohort studies," *Vaccine*, 32(29), pp. 3623–3629. https://doi.org/10.1016/j.vaccine.2014.04.085

UK Health Security Agency (2013) "Surveillance and monitoring for vaccine safety: the green book, chapter 9," *GOV.UK* Available at: https://www.gov.uk/government/publications/surveillance-and-monitoring-for-vaccine-safety-the-green-book-chapter-9

UK Health Security Agency (2015) "Rotavirus: the green book, chapter 27b," *GOV.UK* https://www.gov.uk/government/publications/rotavirus-the-green-book-chapter-27b

UK Health Security Agency (2019) "What to expect after vaccinations," *GOV.UK* Available at: https://www.gov.uk/government/publications/what-to-expect-after-vaccinations

UK Health Security Agency (2020) "Yellow fever: the green book, chapter 35," *GOV.UK* Available at: https://www.gov.uk/government/publications/yellow-fever-the-green-book-chapter-35.

UK Health Security Agency (2022a) "Flu vaccination programme 2022 to 2023: information for healthcare practitioners," *GOV.UK* Available at: https://www.gov.uk/government/publications/flu-vaccination-programme-information-for-healthcare-practitioners

UK Health Security Agency (2022b) "Vaccines and porcine gelatine," *GOV.UK* https://www.gov.uk/government/publications/vaccines-and-porcine-gelatine.

UKHSA (2023). HPV vaccination and cervical cancer information https://www.gov.uk/government/publications/hpv-vaccination-and-cervical-cancer-addressing-the-myths/hpv-vaccination-and-cervical-cancer-information (accessed 22/6/24)

Vesikari, T. *et al.* (2013) "Immunogenicity and safety of an investigational multicomponent, recombinant, meningococcal serogroup B vaccine (4CMenB) administered concomitantly with routine infant and child vaccinations: results of two randomised trials," *The Lancet*, 381(9869), pp. 825–835. https://doi.org/10.1016/s0140-6736(12)61961-8

Wilhelmsen, L. (2002) "Role of the Data and Safety Monitoring Committee (DSMC)," *Statistics in Medicine*, 21(19), pp. 2823–2829. https://doi.org/10.1002/sim.1286

World Health Organization, Mort, Molly, Baleta, Adele, Destefano, Frank, Nsubuga, Jane G. et al. (2013). Vaccine safety basics: learning manual. World Health Organization. https://iris.who.int/handle/10665/340576 (accessed 22/6/24)

World Health Organization (2016) Global manual on surveillance of adverse events following immunization" *www.who.int* Available at: https://www.who.int/publications/i/item/9789241507769 (accessed 21/6/24)

Being a Safe Practitioner

Helen Donovan, Sarah Lang, Ashling Kerr, Lindsey Milroy, and Chris Green

4.1 Introduction

Being a safe practitioner is a fundamental aspect of all clinical practice. Professional registration requires practitioners comply with the standards for their regulating body. For registered nurses and midwives, this means being accountable to the Nursing and Midwifery Council (NMC) and being compliant with the NMC Code (NMC 2023)—other healthcare professionals similarly must comply with their respective regulator. Healthcare support staff while not accountable to a regulator are still accountable for their actions—NHS Scotland has a healthcare support worker code of conduct available via the TURAS platform (TURAS 2009). The public has a legal right to safe and competent care whether the practitioner providing the care is a registered professional or not.

Where standards exist, the practitioners need to be trained to the standard of practice defined and to be assessed as competent to do the work. They also need to have support, such as access to senior staff, the necessary resources and governance processes in place so workers are not expected to work beyond their level of competence and that they have access to education and ongoing continuing professional development, to make sure they can deliver safe care. The education and training of vaccinators is the focus of this chapter, but the principles of accountability and delegation of practice will also be discussed.

H. Donovan (✉)
Specialist in Immunisation and Vaccination, Independent Nurse Consultant, London, UK

S. Lang · C. Green
London, UK

A. Kerr
Public Health Agency Northern Ireland, Belfast, UK

L. Milroy
NHS Education for Scotland, Edinburgh, UK

© Springer Nature Switzerland AG 2025
H. Donovan, H. Bedford (eds.), *Safe Vaccine Administration*,
https://doi.org/10.1007/978-3-031-92498-9_4

The revised guidelines from the National Institute for Health Care Excellence (NICE) recommend that all healthcare professionals who either promote or administer vaccines are trained in accordance with a nationally agreed curriculum (NICE 2022). The National Minimum Standards and Core Curriculum for Vaccination Training, set out the core training requirements for all vaccinators in the UK (UKHSA 2025). The application and use of these in practice will be considered in this chapter.

Practitioners also need to ensure they have appropriate indemnity cover to undertake the work they do. This is to make sure that the cost of any potential future legal action by the patient can be covered. All healthcare workers who are employed by NHS organisations or GP practices will be covered by their employer's indemnity—those employed by other providers should ensure employer indemnity is in place—the NMC has further information on this (NMC 2022).

4.2 Accountability and Delegation

Legally all practitioners, whether they are registered professional practitioners, unregistered support staff or students, are responsible for the care they give. If they make mistakes, while their employer has responsibility, they too can be held liable for the consequences. This means not only do they need to have the required training to undertake the work, but they also need to be assessed as competent and not work beyond their level of competence. This can be challenging as is human nature to want to help and show willingness when asked to do more work by employers or managers.

Similarly, when delegating work to others, an individual is accountable for the decision to delegate and needs to consider the core principles. In summary, the principles vaccinators must consider are as follows (NMC 2020):

- Is delegating this work to others in the best interests of the patients, for example, would not doing it delay them having the vaccines?
- Vaccinators must have the required training and education and feel confident that it is within their scope of competence. For example, staff trained to deliver influenza vaccines should not be delegated to deliver other vaccines without further education and competency assessment.
- Vaccinators must understand their limitations and know who and how to refer to as needed or if problems arise. Support should be immediately accessible to them.
- Vaccinators must also have the appropriate authority to do the work, such as being part of their job description and role. In addition, in the case of giving medicines such as vaccines, this means there is appropriate medicines authorisation in place (Chap. 8 discusses this in detail).
- Is there facility for ongoing evaluation to monitor the outcomes of the work being undertaken and opportunity for reflecting on practice and to access ongoing continuing professional development.
- In accepting delegated work, vaccinators understand their accountability in accepting, to work safely and to the agreed standards.

The National Minimum Standards and Core Curriculum for Vaccination Training (UKHSA 2025) set out additional considerations for training education and support of health care support workers HCSW who are vaccinating. The Northern Ireland Practice and Education Council for Nursing and Midwifery (NIPEC) has a useful tool to support delegation (NIPEC 2024).

See the Appendix "Vaccinators: Best Practice/Scope of Practice Considerations".

4.3 Education for Vaccinators

The standards for immunisation and vaccination training are given in Box 4.1.

> **Box 4.1 Education and Training Standards for Vaccinators**
> - All registered healthcare practitioners working in England, Wales and Northern Ireland UKHSA National Minimum Standards and Core Curriculum for Vaccination Training. National Minimum Standards and Core Curriculum for Immunisation Training for Registered Healthcare Practitioners.
> - Northern Ireland have some additional resource for healthcare support staff who are working to a National Protocol Training Requirements for Non Registered Staff working under the National Protocol (hscni.net).
> - Education resources for staff working in Scotland are aligned to these standards and are available online: NES TURAS Learn.
>
> In addition, there are supplementary standards for those who are solely involved with the influenza or COVID-19 vaccination programmes as it is recognised—they just need to have the specifics related to these programmes.

The revised National Minimum Standards and Core Curriculum for Vaccination Training, set out the core training requirements for all vaccinators in the UK (UKHSA 2025) have evolved since the original publication in 2004. They exist to support the education and training of vaccinators by describing essential knowledge and skills for safe vaccination practice.

They detail the requirement for the following:

1. Foundation or core training for vaccinators who are new to this area of practice
2. Annual updates to make sure vaccinators stay up-to-date

The organisation of vaccination programmes, including education and training, is devolved to the local level (Chantler et al. 2016). The application of the national standards to practice and understanding of them by individuals and organisations is subject to wide variation across the UK. Access to training and the time available for education can be challenging for many vaccinators. It is, however, a core element of the NICE guidelines, and while NICE guidance is for England, the principles apply throughout the UK to support immunisation programmes (NICE 2022).

Successful vaccination programmes are dependent on healthcare practitioners being skilled and well trained to ensure public trust and confidence in the vaccine programme are maintained (NICE evidence review 2022). All healthcare professionals who either promote or administer vaccines are recommended to be trained in accordance with a nationally agreed curriculum (NICE 2022). The National Minimum Standards and Core Curriculum for Vaccination Training are applicable for all vaccinators UKHSA (2025). The application and utility of these in practice will be considered in this chapter.

There has been a fundamental shift over the last 40 years, from vaccine administration being the responsibility of doctors and in some cases health visitors (Peckham et al., 1989) to it now being seen as a core nursing role with nursing and midwifery staff responsible for most vaccine service delivery for the population in the United Kingdom. Other professional groups, particularly pharmacy teams, are also increasingly involved. As this book is aimed primarily for nursing and midwifery staff, they are the focus but the core principles apply to anyone delivering vaccine services.

Safe vaccination practice involves more than simply administering a vaccine. As described in the other chapters in the book, the UK vaccination programme is complex and constantly evolving and developing. Alongside this, public concerns and perceptions about vaccines are also affected by media messages and increasingly social media. Vaccinators need to be well informed and keep up-to-date to be able to discuss vaccination with people.

Multicomponent studies which include immunisation training for healthcare workers have been shown to improve vaccine uptake (Crocker-Buque et al. 2017). Attitudinal surveys conducted to explore people's attitudes to vaccination invariably cite healthcare professionals as the key most trusted sources of information and in influencing vaccine decisions (UKHSA 2023, Sherman et al. 2023)—this obviously necessitates they are appropriately trained and have continued education. Confident communication is essential—the evidence shows that when staff have had training, they report being more confident having conversations and giving advice on vaccination (Vishram et al. 2018).

It is also clear that staff need to be able to tailor their approach depending on the needs of the community, whether this is the age, ethnicity or wider demographics of the population being served (NIHR 2023)—this is discussed further in Chap. 12. Ensuring vaccinators are appropriately trained is essential to the continued success of the UK vaccination programme.

Vaccines are medicinal products, and safe administration involves thorough understanding of who can and can't safely receive them. This assessment is usually made by the person administering the vaccine but may on occasion be undertaken by a registered healthcare professional such as a nurse, doctor or pharmacist and then delegated to a healthcare support worker to administer the vaccine. The principles of delegation as discussed earlier must be considered, and further medicines management legislation in respect of this is also discussed in Chap. 8.

4.4 Varying Learning Needs of Vaccinators

The vaccination workforce has a broad range of learning needs largely prescribed by the part of the programme they are delivering, their role and the context of their workplace. For many, vaccination is part of a range of much wider responsibilities for the individual nurse, and they may not be afforded sufficient time for vaccination training and education, and it may not be considered a priority when seen against all the other work and continuing professional development needs. Depending on the area of work, the learning needs will also vary, for example, as nurses working in primary care or in immunisation and vaccination teams in the community deliver vaccinations across the life course, their learning needs encompass many programmes and large sections of the population. Those working in schools will be working with specific population groups but will also need to work in a variety of settings and be able to liaise effectively with education providers.

Having the skills and competence to be able to talk with people and groups in different areas and across different age groups requires vaccinators to draw on a range of knowledge and skills so they can effectively tailor messages and information.

As discussed elsewhere in this book, change is inherent to vaccine programmes, and the UK vaccine programmes have become far more complex over the last 30 years including the types of vaccines used and the populations receiving them (Lang et al. 2020a; Lang et al. 2020b). The vaccination workforce needs to be informed through continuing professional development to ensure they can manage changes efficiently and safely. How vaccinators can achieve this is discussed further in this chapter.

4.5 Learning and Skills Acquisition

The core curriculum sets out the key topic areas that all vaccinators need to have. Safe and effective vaccination requires more than just the theoretical learning about the vaccines, the vaccine preventable diseases and the processes for safe administration. It requires the vaccinator to develop practice and understanding of the needs of the individuals and populations they are working with. It also necessitates that they recognise their own background experiences and therefore learning needs.

Core knowledge: This is explicit in the national core curriculum content. It includes having knowledge about the vaccines and how they work, the vaccine preventable diseases and the practical processes for safe administration, reporting adverse reactions UKHSA (2025). This document provides clear standards for training.

Cultural knowledge and awareness: This is less easy to define and generally developed through experience of life and work. It is necessary for the general setup and management of the service and communication and consultation skills. These will often be acquired through experience and practice. This art and skill is learnt largely through working with others and supervised practice and reflecting on practice in a work-based setting (see Box 4.1 for practice reflection for skills acquisition).

Personal knowledge: This includes the beliefs and feelings that individuals bring to their learning and how they use knowledge. It might include a nurse with no specific paediatric training being anxious about vaccinating children. It could also be an individual's own beliefs about the value of a specific vaccine.

Personal knowledge is an important consideration—it can influence how additional knowledge is assimilated.

Box 4.2 provides a reflective example to guide people through these processes.

Box 4.2 Reflection: Skills Acquisition

Consider how your vaccine consultations are structured and delivered or for school or mass vaccination scenario how are they set up:

- Is the service friendly and accessible, particularly where people have learning needs?
- Do people have privacy to ask questions?
- Is it easy for people to understand where to go?
- Are staff roles clearly identified?

Consider how you do things and then why you do them that way?

Is it because that's how you were taught, or is it the cultural practices within your workplace?

Are new staff with up-to-date information encouraged to bring up-to-date information back to more experienced staff to support practice.

The way things are done in a workplace can significantly impact the success of the vaccine programme.

It is imperative that all organisations and employers provide their vaccinator workforce with the time to access education and training and give time to develop their skills and knowledge.

How individuals use the core theoretical knowledge is influenced by their cultural and personal knowledge, experience and beliefs. Knowing something doesn't always relate to application in practice. The art and skill of vaccination practice is learnt largely through working with others and supervised practice in a work-based setting. A period of supervised practice is recommended in the core curriculum. The National Minimum Standards and Core Curriculum for Vaccination Training (UKHSA 2025), include a comprehensive competency tool which has been designed to support this, and while it can be completed by the individual on their own, it is probably best done jointly with a supervisor in practice such as a line manager or more experienced colleague with the necessary skills and experience. The RCN Immunisation Knowledge and Skills Competence Assessment Tool (RCN 2022) is similarly designed to support this. Immunisation Knowledge and Skills Competence Assessment Tool (RCN 2022).

Work based learning, with supervision and support while doing the job can be tailored to support vaccinators development this and ongoing continuing professional development will be discussed later in the chapter.

4.6 Becoming a Vaccinator: Foundation Training

The national standards for vaccination training stipulate that specific foundation training must be undertaken by those new to vaccination practice and that these individuals are assessed as competent by an appropriate registered practitioner who is itself skilled and up-to-date in vaccination practice UKHSA (2025). The following are recommended for foundation training:

1. "Theoretical" foundation training through either face to face or e-learning or a combination of both. The document describes the core curriculum requirements with explicit learning outcomes for each.
2. Work-based learning through supervised practice—this is an essential component and often overlooked. It can help to use the learning outcomes for each element to inform how best to maximise work-based learning. A competency assessment tool is included within the standards (UKHSA 2025). Also, the use of the RCN competency development tool (RCN 2022) similarly can be used.
3. Evidence of competence. This is often a certificate of attendance, but this alone of course does not demonstrate evidence of competence. Vaccinators should reflect on both the theoretical and practical work-based learning.

Vaccinators require time and support to develop their skills in the workplace. An assumption is often made that once theoretical foundation training has been completed, a learner returns to the workplace and puts that knowledge to work as taught. What is taught on a study day doesn't always take account of the learning that may occur through the connection of individuals, mediation of knowledge through cultural tools and artefacts and how different contexts utilise different forms of knowledge use and application. The danger of such an assumption is that it takes no account of the cultural and personal aspects of learning as discussed earlier and considers theory and practice knowledge movement as a linear process.

What does this mean in practice? An illustrative example is described in Box 4.3.

Box 4.3 Practice Example to Illustrate Theory Practice Reflection

Sarah is a new PN who recently attended a 2-day foundation vaccination course. On this course, she was taught the rationale for the pertussis vaccination in pregnancy programme and felt she had really understood it and believed strongly in the importance of it.

Sarah was well supported with her work-based learning, and during a supervised session with her mentor, a pregnant woman attended for her pertussis vaccination. Sarah took the lead in talking to the woman but didn't find it very easy to explain to her why she should have the pertussis vaccine. Whilst she did successfully obtain consent Sarah identified that she needed to practice her explanation and draw on some of the communication skills she had also been taught about framing messages and exploring concerns.

(continued)

> **Box 4.3** (continued)
> This is an example of how knowledge is recontextualised into the workplace—Sarah knew the facts but she hadn't worked out how to explain them clearly to a patient. Vaccinators sometimes refer to the way they explain things as their 'patter'—and they become second nature with time and experience. Sarah needed to try using her knowledge, reflect on it.

The goal of core or foundation training is for the vaccinator to be signed off as competent to safely administer vaccines or provide advice about vaccinations.

A competency assessment tool is recommended to support this and can be used in a number of ways:

- Self-assessment by the vaccinator
- Identification of learning needs
- To facilitate discussion between the supervising clinician and the vaccinator
- Agreeing training programmes
- Guiding next steps

Theoretical training should include how new vaccinators can develop competence using the tool. Anecdotal reports from vaccinators suggest supervised practice and use of the competency tool is widely adopted in practice.

Organisations providing vaccination services should include evidence of competency assessment completion within its governance responsibilities and ensure that when training new vaccinators, adequate supervision and time is made available.

Completion of core or fundamental training including assessment of their competency and sign off, enables them to practice independently, vaccinator learning and education and continuing professional development is ongoing.

4.7 Continuing Professional Development: Keeping Up-to-Date

Being up-to-date is part of professional registration and also part of the quality assurance of the programme/workforce, and each workplace should have appropriate governance arrangements to oversee this.

The core curriculum recommends vaccinators should be able to demonstrate how they have kept up-to-date on an annual basis.

As stated, vaccine programmes continually evolve and develop. Vaccinators must be able to evidence how they have kept up-to-date with the current schedule and any changes to vaccination practice. Where there are changes updates may in fact need to be more frequent. How individual practitioners achieve this is ultimately up to them but needs to be done in a way which supports their own professional practice needs. Updates may be in the form of taught sessions or online courses or webinars but could be other self-directed learning, identified by the individual vaccinator as their learning needs—ideas for achieving this are given later in the chapter on how to keep up-to-date.

4.7.1 Identifying Learning Needs

Vaccinators have a range of skills and knowledge, with some areas/topics of strength and some areas they may be less confident in. Vaccinators can target learning to meet their own individual needs—but how do they identify these? Here are some examples:

- Reflection in or on an event
- In response to a critical incident or error
- Self-assessing against a criterion such as the NMS competency assessment tool or learning objectives
- In response to feedback from peer, manager or patient

Box 4.4 provides a practice example to demonstrate this type of reflection on action.

> **Box 4.4 Practice Example Reflection on Practice**
> An experienced practice nurse is very happy and confident vaccinating infants but finds vaccinating pre-school aged children challenging. They share their thoughts with a colleague and are interested to hear how their colleague utilises distraction techniques to support vaccination of pre-school aged children. The practice nurse reflects on their own practice and identifies that distraction is something they don't know much about and decides to learn more through web searches and further reading. The practice nurse documents what they have learnt from their reading and reflects on how they will use this in practice in the future.

4.7.2 Activities for Keeping Up-to-Date

This is ultimately personal to each individual and should be based on identified learning needs. While many people appreciate taught update sessions, these may not completely meet all the learning needs and may not always be easily available.

Table 4.1 presents a number of suggestions for how vaccinators can keep up-to-date utilising currently available resources.

Some suggestions focus on individual learning, while others focus on learning with peers/other team members. Learning is not an isolated activity, and creating and taking opportunities to learn with others is important.

Whichever method is used to update, it is essential to document the learning from the activity. A certificate of attendance demonstrates attendance at an event rather than the learning and how this will impact individual practice (see Table 4.1 for examples).

Vaccinators are encouraged to utilise a range of methods and managers/employers to take the time to explore reflective accounts.

Table 4.1 Activities to support keeping up-to-date

Activity	Further suggestions
Vaccine update Register to receive "'Vaccine Update" (https://www.gov.uk/government/collections/vaccine-update) or the Public Health Scotland equivalent which colleagues can also register to receive via email Show all releases—Publications—Public Health Scotland Read regularly and access the hyperlinks and documents	Disseminate vaccine update to colleagues Discuss routinely at team meeting—include as a standing agenda item and note key issues discussed in the meeting minutes
Self-briefing and review of information Be up-to-date with national immunisation information England UKHSA immunisation collection portal (https://www.gov.uk/government/collections/immunisation) Northern Ireland Public Health Agency (https://www.publichealth.hscni.net/directorate-public-health/health-protection/immunisationvaccine-preventable-diseases) Scotland Public Health Scotland (https://www.healthscotland.scot/health-topics/immunisation) Wales Public Health Wales (https://phw.nhs.wales/topics/immunisation-and-vaccines/) • Spend time navigating and checking for updates to programmes • Spend time navigating and checking the Green Book	Share new tools with colleagues Arrange a discussion group to review new documents together and take a common approach **Flu vaccination example** Practice team reviews the resources for forthcoming flu season Note key changes to the programme Reflect on complex and patient safety issues Identify patients who do not attend and plan strategies Consider challenges such as safe vaccine storage and ordering
Extend understanding of policy: Read the JCVI minutes • Published three times a year (https://www.gov.uk/government/groups/joint-committee-on-vaccination-and-immunisation)	Identify further journal articles to read referenced within the minutes If the full minutes are too daunting, consider choosing a programme to follow through each meeting
Conferences Conferences may be specific to vaccination programmes or focused on disease areas that are part of the programme	Use learning and feedback from conferences with peers and other team members
Journal articles Identify and read journal articles Set up a journal club to review articles as a group	Identify further reading within the journal articles If you have particular area of practice, consider writing a blog or journal article around this

(continued)

Table 4.1 (continued)

Activity	Further suggestions
Immunology How vaccines work is part of foundation training—this is worth revisiting again when updating	Access the UKHSA immunology animation at immunology for immunisers animation and E learning core modules available at Immunisation—elearning for healthcare (e-lfh.org.uk) Promoting Effective Immunisation Practice: Promoting Effective Immunisation Practice (PEIP) | Turas | Learn (nhs.scot)
Disease epidemiology Vaccine preventable disease epidemiology changes, and the latest data is published by the UKHSA	Access the UKHSA Health Protection Reports for immunisation https://www.gov.uk/government/collections/health-protection-report-latest-infection-reports#immunisation Public Health Scotland for Scottish data: Infectious diseases—Health protection—Our areas of work—Public Health Scotland
Supporting vaccine acceptance There are various tools available here The Oxford Vaccine Knowledge website (https://vaccineknowledge.ox.ac.uk/home) independent, evidence-based information about vaccines and infectious diseases Jitsu vax (Welcome—Jitsuvax) resource designed to support learning to enhance vaccine uptake and knowledge among healthcare professionals and the public See also infographic from NHS Scotland: Improving confidence in vaccines (Improving confidence in vaccines a guide to framing conversations | Turas | Learn (nhs.scot))	Use with colleagues to support reflection with challenging practice scenarios Consider international resources US Centers for Disease Control and Prevention (CDC) The World Health Organization (WHO) Children's Hospital of Philadelphia Vaccine Education Center Australian, sharing knowledge about immunisation SKAI to note that the vaccine schedules and programmes will vary in other countries
Other resources Within this book, there are links to many websites and resources. See the resources section The UKHSA YouTube channel includes a number of resources on vaccines and wider infectious diseases including links to conference and webinar recordings (https://www.youtube.com/channel/UCoFX8yfaEwXNEu3HgLdfomQ)	

4.7.3 Reflection

Reflection is not confined only to the formal types of learning above but on any situation that occurs whether you are a new or experienced vaccinator. Reflection considers the learning either from or during an event and supports practitioners to consider past, present and future actions.

Recording reflections, for example, through logs, provides an opportunity to capture individual learning from activities or practice. Vaccination practice can be challenging and sometimes stressful and often involve emotions. Reflective practice is a useful tool to support the continued development of vaccinators (RCN 2004).

For new vaccinators, a reflective log may be a useful tool in supporting the development of new skills. Logs could include the following:

- Capturing new skill use.
- Considering the emotional impact of being a vaccinator, e.g. some new vaccinators find it difficult to vaccinate babies or giving multiple vaccines to a 12-month-old—exploring the emotional side of vaccination practice is important.
- Evidencing your journey from novice to competent practitioner.
- Planning learning activities with a mentor/supervising practitioner.

Reflection is not just limited to those new to vaccination practice and can be more widely applied. Vaccination practice aligns with all parts of the NMC Code of Conduct by prioritising people, practising effectively, preserving safety and promoting professionalism and trust.

The RCN has a useful resource (Revalidation requirements: Reflection and reflective discussion)—it explores reflection as a revalidation requirement but also as tool for supporting practice.

4.8 Conclusion

Safe practice and the quality of the UK vaccination programme rely on a well-trained and skilled workforce. For vaccinators, this begins with foundation training, both theoretical and workplace supervised practice, leading to a formal competency assessment and continues with update training throughout their career.

The responsibility for education and learning for vaccinators extends from individual practitioners to managers to organisational development leads to education providers and policymakers. Lack of engagement with education and learning for vaccinators is unsatisfactory within any of these groups, and barriers to education must be removed. Governance mechanisms should be utilised to assure the education and skills of the workforce.

References

Chantler T, Lwembe S, Saliba V, Raj T, Mays N, Ramsay M, Mournier Jack S, (2016). "It's a complex mesh"- how large-scale health system reorganisation affected the delivery of the immunisation programme in England: a qualitative study. BMC Health Services Research https://bmchealthservres.biomedcentral.com/articles/10.1186/s12913-016-1711-0 [Accessed October 2023].

Crocker-Buque, T., Edelstein, M. and Mounier-Jack, S., 2017. Interventions to reduce inequalities in vaccine uptake in children and adolescents aged< 19 years: a systematic review. *J Epidemiol Community Health*, *71*(1), pp.87-97.

Lang S, Loving S, McCarthy ND, *et al (2020a)* Two centuries of immunisation in the UK (part 1) *Archives of Disease in Childhood* **105:**115-121.

Lang S, Loving S, McCarthy ND, et al (2020b). Two centuries of immunisation in the UK (part II) *Archives of disease in childhood*, *105*(3), pp.216-222.

NICE (2022). Vaccine uptake in the general population NICE guideline [NG218]Published: 17 May 2022 https://www.nice.org.uk/guidance/ng218 [Accessed October 2023]

NIHR (2023). Promoting vaccination: the right approach for the right group. PUBLIC HEALTH 24.07.23 https://doi.org/10.3310/nihrevidence_59296

NIPEC (2024) Northern Ireland Practice and Education Council for Nursing and Midwifery Delegation tool Delegation | NIPEC (hscni.net) [Accessed June 2024]

NMC (2023) NMC The Code Professional standards of practice and behaviour for nurses, midwives and nursing associates https://www.nmc.org.uk/standards/code/ [Accessed October 2023]

NMC (2020). NMC the Code in action https://www.nmc.org.uk/standards/code/code-in-action/ [Accessed October 2023]

NMC (2022). NMC Professional indemnity arrangement on line https://www.nmc.org.uk/registration/joining-the-register/professional-indemnity-arrangement/ [Accessed October 2023]

RCN (2022) Immunisation Knowledge and Skills Competence Assessment Tool https://www.rcn.org.uk/Professional-Development/publications/immunisation-knowledge-and-skills-competence-assessment-tool-uk-pub-010-074 [Accessed October 2023]

RCN (2004) Resource Revalidation requirements: Reflection and reflective discussion [Accessed June 2024]

Peckham C, Bedford H, Senturia Y. (1989). The Peckham report: National immunisation study: factors influencing immunisation uptake in childhood. Institute of Child Health, London: Horsham: Action research for the crippled child.1989

Sherman S, Lingley-Heath N, Lai J, Sim J, Bedford H, (2023). Parental acceptance of and preferences for administration of routine varicella vaccination in the UK: A study to inform policy. Vaccine 41(8) p 1438-1446. https://doi.org/10.1016/j.vaccine.2023.01.027 Elsevier. [Accessed October 2023]

TURAS (2009) Health Care Support Worker Code of Conduct https://learn.nes.nhs.scot/72181

UKHSA (2023). Childhood vaccines: parental attitudes survey 2022 findings Childhood vaccines: parental attitudes survey 2022 findings - GOV.UK (www.gov.uk) [Accessed October 2023]

UKHSA (2025). National Minimum Standards and Core Curriculum for Vaccination Training https://www.gov.uk/government/publications/national-minimum-standards-and-core-curriculum-for-immunisation-training-for-registered-healthcare-practitioners

Vishram B, Letley L, Van Hoek AJ, Silverton L, Donovan H, Adams C Green D, Edwards A Yarwood J Bedford H Amirthalingam G Cambell H 2018. Vaccination in pregnancy: Attitudes of nurses, midwives and health visitors in England. Human Vaccines & immunotherapeutics. 14:1,179–188 https://doi.org/10.1080/21645515.2017.1382789

Vaccine Storage: "The Cold Chain"

5

Laura Craig and Michelle Falconer

5.1 Introduction

Vaccines protect against disease and prevent death but can only do so if their potency is retained from the point of manufacture until the vaccine is administered to the patient. As vaccines are biological products, they are susceptible to extreme temperatures and light, and so they have specific storage requirements and a limited shelf life. For these reasons, to avoid compromising the quality of the vaccine, it is essential that all vaccines are stored and transported under the correct conditions.

Vaccine manufacturers are responsible for providing information about the storage conditions their vaccines require to maintain potency for the duration of their shelf life. This information is published in their Summary of Product Characteristics (SmPC) which can be found on the electronic medicines compendium website (www.medicines.org.uk/emc/) as well as inside the vaccine packaging.

5.2 Cold Chain Overview

- All vaccines used in the UK are recommended to be transported and stored within the temperature range specified by the manufacturer. For most vaccines, this range is +2 °C to +8 °C. This is known as the "cold chain", and an excursion outside the recommended temperature range is known as a cold chain breach.
- For this reason, vaccines need to be kept in a purpose built, carefully monitored and well-maintained vaccine or medicines fridge.

L. Craig (✉)
Lead Immunisation Nurse Specialist Immunisation Programmes: Design, Implementation and Clinical Guidance Division, UK Health Security Agency, London, UK
e-mail: Laura.Craig@ukhsa.gov.uk

M. Falconer
Public Health Scotland (PHS), Edinburgh, UK

© Springer Nature Switzerland AG 2025
H. Donovan, H. Bedford (eds.), *Safe Vaccine Administration*,
https://doi.org/10.1007/978-3-031-92498-9_5

- Regular reading and recording of the fridge temperature needs to be conducted, ideally twice a day: at the start of the working day before any vaccines are administered and at the end of the working day to ensure a record of the fridge temperature is available should there be any temperature breach or issue with the power supply overnight.
- Where vaccination is taking place off-site, for example, in a school or a patient's home, the vaccines should be placed and transported in a temperature monitored cool box intended for vaccine transportation. Vaccine storage recommendations should continue to be followed, including regular monitoring and recording of the temperature. Any unused vaccines can then be returned to the fridge and used for subsequent immunisation sessions as long as it has been documented that the temperature in the cool box was maintained within the recommended range (UKHSA 2017b).

5.3 Factors Affecting Vaccine Stability

Potency can be affected by prolonged exposure of the vaccine to both warm and to freezing temperatures. Some vaccines are more stable than others (World Health Organisation (WHO) 2006), and the effect of a cold chain breach on a vaccine's potency can vary depending upon the type of vaccine, the temperature and the length of time it was stored at that temperature.

For example,

- Live attenuated vaccines tend to be more susceptible to extremes of heat than inactivated vaccines (Fredman and Kroger n.d., General Immunization Practices Chap. 10).
- Inactivated vaccines containing aluminium as an adjuvant can be permanently damaged by freezing.

Any exposures to temperatures outside the recommended +2 °C to +8 °C range should be considered to be potentially damaging, and a risk assessment should be completed before using the vaccines involved. Any previous exposures outside the recommended range should also be considered along with the incident itself as each exposure has a cumulative effect on vaccine potency.

5.4 Impact of Incorrect Storage on Vaccines

Incorrect storage of vaccines can lead to vaccine wastage if vaccines need to be disposed of. This is expensive for the NHS and can also directly impact on patient confidence in the vaccination programme if they have to be recalled for revaccination.

5 Vaccine Storage: "The Cold Chain"

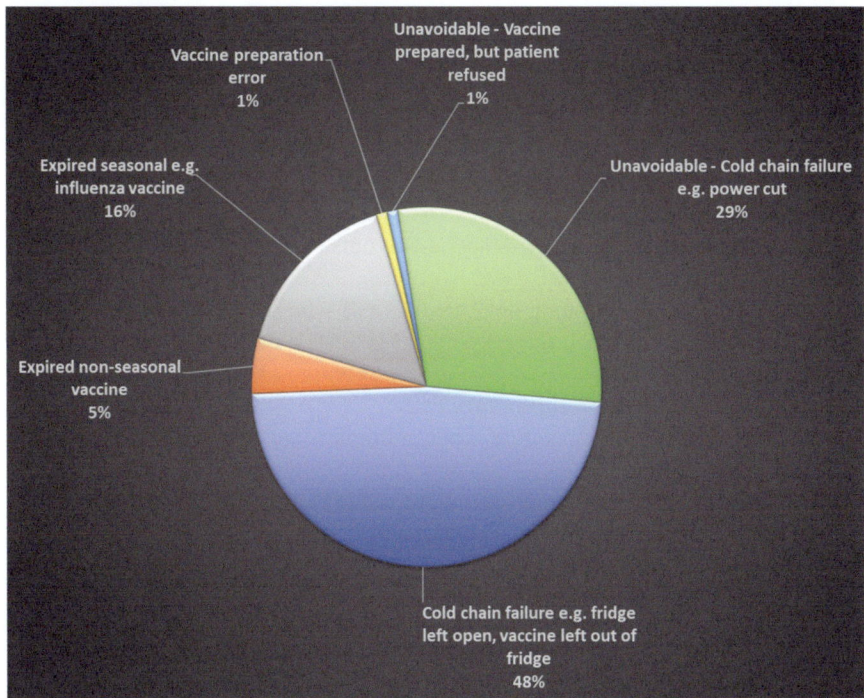

Fig. 5.1 Causes of vaccine wastage incidents reported through ImmForm (2023) (figure published on ImmForm and obtained from the UKHSA vaccine team, chapter authors, who collected the data and created the pie chart permission to use it)

The consequences of incorrect vaccine storage can be high in terms of both the financial cost of vaccines that then have to be discarded and in terms of the potential for them to result in failure to evoke the required immune response for patients which may lead to them requiring revaccination or potentially developing the disease that they thought they were protected against.

Information relating to vaccine wastage is collected by the UK Health Security Agency (UKHSA) using the online ImmForm vaccine ordering and reporting system.

Figure 5.1 shows the causes of vaccine wastage incidents reported via ImmForm for 2023. In this year alone, vaccine wastage incidents reported due to both avoidable and unavoidable incidents had a list price value of £5.8 million. This is potentially an under-reporting of vaccine wastage.

The majority of the unavoidable cold chain failures were due to power cuts (£1.66 million of the total). However, most of the total value of vaccine wastage was caused by avoidable incidents (70.3%, £4.1 million). Wastage caused by fridge malfunctions, fridge door left open or vaccine left out of fridge was the largest contributory factor (£2.8 million).

5.5 Causes of Vaccine Wastage

The most commonly reported reasons for avoidable cold chain incidents (UKHSA 2016, 2017a, 2019, 2023) include the following:

- Vaccines being stored outside of the recommended temperature range of +2 °C to +8 °C
- No action being taken when temperatures outside of the recommended range were observed and recorded
- Temperature recording being delegated to staff who do not understand the correct procedure to follow if the temperature is outside of the recommended range
- Overstocking of fridges
- Failing to record fridge temperatures daily
- Failing to reset the temperature when minimum and maximum temperatures have been recorded
- Setting the fridge temperature too high resulting in the temperature frequently exceeding the recommended 8 °C maximum
- Fridge door left open
- Fridge being accidently switched off
- Broken fridge or lack of adequate equipment

Table 5.1 provides a summary of the recommended actions needed to prevent or minimise future vaccine wastage.

Table 5.1 Avoidable reasons for vaccine wastage and suggested actions to mitigate against wastage

Avoidable reason for vaccine wastage	Action to take to prevent vaccine wastage
Fridge door left open	• Ensure the seal on the door is intact • Ensure that each person who uses the fridge checks that the door is closed after use • Use the lock if there is one fitted
Fridge accidently switched off	• Wire the fridge into a switchless socket (preferably) • Alternatively, put a "do not unplug" label on the plug
Equipment failure (not as a result of power failure)	• Ensure fridge and related items such as thermometer and data logger are serviced and calibrated yearly or in accordance with the manufacturer's instructions • Ensure that there is a process for routinely checking that the data logger is functioning and batteries are replaced before they wear out
Wrong temperature range/lack of temperature monitoring	• Fridge temperature should be set to run at 5 °C • Designated person or deputy to record and document the temperature at the start and end of each day • Person recording the temperature to immediately inform designated person of any temperature outside the recommended range so that corrective action can be taken as soon as possible

(continued)

Table 5.1 (continued)

Avoidable reason for vaccine wastage	Action to take to prevent vaccine wastage
Lack of or inadequate equipment	• Review vaccine needs based on patient population, and ensure sufficient fridge capacity so that the fridge is not overcrowded • Consider times of additional demand on fridge capacity such as during flu vaccination "season"
Stock left out of fridge or prepared but damaged, lost or mislaid before use	• Check vaccine deliveries and place in fridge immediately • Notify designated person or deputy of delivery when stock is received. Ensure reception staff are aware of the importance of doing this and that they make it a priority • Prepare vaccines during the patient consultation, not in advance
Wrong vaccine being ordered	• Implement a vaccine stock management system and review it before placing vaccine orders
Vaccine expiring before it could be used/excess stock being ordered	• Hold no more than 2–4 weeks' supply of vaccines and review scheduled clinics before placing vaccine orders • Use stock with shortest expiry date first • Ensure staff understand post thaw expiry dates for vaccines that were previously stored frozen

5.6 National Recommendations for Vaccine Storage, Distribution and Disposal and Vaccine Incidents

A key recommendation for ensuring good vaccine storage systems are in place is to designate a named lead and a deputy within each organisation to be responsible for the ordering and management of vaccines and their storage.

All those involved in the ordering, storage or administration of vaccines should be familiar with the national recommendations for vaccine storage, distribution and disposal. These are published in the "Storage, Distribution and Disposal of Vaccines" chapter in the online edition of the Green Book (n.d.) (which contains information relating to the following:

- Storage requirements for vaccines
- Ways of obtaining centrally purchased vaccines
- Recommendations for stock management
- Safe disposal of expired or damaged vaccines

If vaccines are exposed to temperatures outside of the recommended range, a risk assessment should be conducted before either discarding them or using them. The risk assessment should consider the following:

- Temperature the vaccines have been exposed to
- Duration of that exposure
- Likely impact of it on the effectiveness of the vaccine

Information on the likely impact of the storage temperatures on the vaccines can be obtained from the vaccine manufacturer. Any affected vaccines should be quarantined within the recommended temperature range until that information has been obtained and a decision regarding future use of the vaccines has been made. No vaccine or vaccine storage equipment should be discarded until the incident has been discussed with the local Screening and Immunisation Team (SIT).

The safe transport, storage and handling of vaccines is recognised as a essential component of a safe and efficient immunisation service, as outlined in the Quality criteria for an effective immunisation programme (UKHSA 2025). The UKHSA (2022) publication *Vaccine Incident Guidance* or, in Scotland, the Public Health Scotland publication *Guidance on Vaccine Storage and Handling* can be used to inform any local risk assessment. The "vaccine storage incident checklist" provided at the end of the guidance document (or any locally provided equivalent) should be fully completed so that there is comprehensive information on which to base any decisions.

Any vaccine wastage should be reported using the online stock incident form available on ImmForm by following the guidance in their "fridge failures and stock incidents" help sheet.

5.7 Vaccine Incident Scenario

Box 5.1 describes a vaccine storage incident and the considerable cost, not just financial but also in terms of staff time, alongside the considerable risks to vaccine confidence that a vaccine incident poses.

> **Box 5.1 Cold Chain Scenario**
> A Care Quality Commission (CQC) inspection visit at the *Needles GP surgery* revealed that the temperature recordings of a vaccine fridge had been out of the recommended range of +2 °C to +8 °C on several occasions in the preceding 3 months. Although a member of the practice team had been delegated the task of recording the fridge temperatures twice a day, no training had been given so when deviations from the recommended range occurred, no corrective action was taken. The minimum temperature had been recorded as -1 °C on five consecutive days.
>
> The practice nurse reported this to their local Screening and Immunisation team (SIT) and was advised to investigate the incident further by
>
> 1. Confirming with the responsible member of staff that they had used the correct procedure for recording the fridge temperature and that they had reset it after each reading
>   – *This had been done but no action taken.*
> 2. Monitoring the fridge temperature using a data logger for 48 h
>   – *This revealed that the temperature was reaching −1 °C.*
> 3. Arranging for an inspection from a fridge engineer
>   – *This confirmed the fridge was faulty and needed replacement.*
>
> (continued)

Box 5.1 (continued)

4. Requesting vaccine stability information from the manufacturers for vaccines in the fridge
   – *to establish whether the potency of any of the vaccines was considered to be compromised by exposure to temperatures below 0 °C*

- A local incident team was formed—the Practice Nurse discarded all compromised stock and completed an ImmForm vaccine wastage report. This highlighted an indicative cost of wasted vaccines of almost £5000.
- As there was no back-up fridge or storage option, all scheduled immunisation appointments were cancelled and rebooked. The surgery had to install and set up a new fridge and order replacement stock, before recommencing vaccination clinics.
- Recipients of vaccines whose potency was deemed to have been compromised were identified, and a revaccination schedule was developed for each recipient.
- A communication plan was also developed, and information resources for patients and a response for potential media interest were prepared.

The patient review revealed the following:

Twenty-eight infants, four pre-school aged children and three adolescents had received one or more doses of a potentially compromised vaccine. Seven patients had received travel vaccines.

- Letters were sent out to parents and patients informing them of the storage incident and the reason for offering an additional dose of vaccine. Not all of them accepted the offer of revaccination and therefore remained potentially susceptible to the infection. Some were upset to learn that the vaccines had not been more carefully stored and monitored.
- Two of the revaccinated children developed a local reaction to the additional dose of vaccine, but otherwise the repeat doses of vaccine were well tolerated.
- The incident was resource intensive and affected patients' overall confidence in the surgery.

As a result, the practice

- Ensured that all their staff had received cold chain training
- Instigated regular audits of their cold chain practice
- Ensured that the vaccine fridge was regularly serviced, that alarms were correctly set and that a data logger was installed
- Advised other local practices of the potential consequences of vaccine cold chain incidents

5.8 Conclusion

Vaccines save lives, protect against disease and help to fight antimicrobial resistance, but to ensure that they do so, they must always be stored and transported within the recommended temperature range of +2 °C to +8 °C.

The potency of vaccines that are exposed to temperatures outside of this range may be compromised, and a risk assessment should be conducted before discarding any vaccines or administering them to patients.

Nearly half of all vaccine wastage occurs for avoidable reasons, and simple actions can be implemented to minimise or prevent these from occurring. Vaccinators have a responsibility not to waste vaccines by ensuring they adhere to good practice recommendations on vaccine storage.

Key Resources
Green book Chap. 3: Storage, distribution and disposal of vaccines available at https://www.gov.uk/government/publications/storage-distribution-and-disposal-of-vaccines-the-green-book-chapter-3

The ImmForm website available at https://portal.immform.dh.gov.uk/Logon.aspx?returnurl=%2f

Vaccine handling and protocols published by UKHSA Including

- Vaccine incident guidance: responding to vaccine errors available at https://www.gov.uk/government/publications/vaccine-incident-guidance-responding-to-vaccine-errors
- Off label vaccine leaflets available at www.gov.uk/government/publications/off-label-vaccineleaflets
    - Off label vaccines: an introductory guide for healthcare professionals
    - Off label vaccines: a guide for parents
- 'Guidance on the use of vaccines that have been temporarily stored outside of the recommended temperature range' leaflet available at www.gov.uk/government/publications/vaccines-stored-outside-the-recommended-temperature-rangeleaflet
- 'Keep your vaccines healthy' poster and magnet available to order available at www.gov.uk/government/publications/keep-your-vaccines-healthy-poster

Guidance on vaccine storage and handling published by PHS available at HPS Website - Guidance on Vaccine Storage and Handling (scot.nhs.uk)

Electronic medicines compendium available at https://www.medicines.org.uk/emc/.

e learning for health online immunisation course, vaccine storage module, available at https://www.e-lfh.org.uk/programmes/immunisation/

References

Fredman M.S, Kroger A.T. (n.d.) General Immunization Practices (Chapter 10) in Orenstein WA, Offit PA, Edwards KM, Plotkin SA. Plotkin's Vaccines. 8th Edition. Elsevier

UKHSA. Immunisation against infectious disease (the Green book), storage, distribution and disposal of vaccines (chapter 3), available at www.gov.uk/government/publications/storage-distribution-and-disposal-of-vaccines-the-green-book-chapter-3

UKHSA. (2022) Vaccine Incident Guidance: Responding to errors in vaccine storage, handling and administration (last updated 2022), available at https://www.gov.uk/government/publications/vaccine-incident-guidance-responding-to-vaccine-errors

UKHSA. (2025) Guidance: Quality criteria for an effective immunisation programme https://www.gov.uk/government/publications/quality-criteria-for-an-effective-immunisation-programme (07/07/2025)

UKHSA. Vaccine Update issue 242 (March 2016) Cold chain, how are we doing. https://assets.publishing.service.gov.uk/government/uploads/system/uploads/attachment_data/file/510376/PHE_9750_VU_242_March_2016_03_web.pdf

UKHSA Vaccine update issue 269 (August 2017a) CQC findings: Immunisation in primary care https://assets.publishing.service.gov.uk/government/uploads/system/uploads/attachment_data/file/643758/VU_269_August_2017.pdf

UKHSA, Vaccine update issue 271 (October 2017b) Interpretation of vaccine storage requirements Available at https://assets.publishing.service.gov.uk/government/uploads/system/uploads/attachment_data/file/653401/VU_271_october_2017.pdf

UKHSA, Vaccine update issue 297 (July 2019) Vaccine wastage, time to check your fridges! Available at https://assets.publishing.service.gov.uk/government/uploads/system/uploads/attachment_data/file/820795/PHE_vaccine_update_297_July_2019.pdf

UKHSA, Vaccine Update: issue 338 (May 2023). Vaccine wastage. https://www.gov.uk/government/publications/vaccine-update-issue-338-may-2023/vaccine-update-issue-338-may-2023 (accessed 27/6/24)

World Health Organisation (WHO) Temperature sensitivity of vaccines (2006), available at https://apps.who.int/iris/bitstream/handle/10665/69387/WHO_IVB_06.10_eng.pdf;jsessionid=11564C53F0ED539339A6414DB27606B7?sequence=1

Discussing Vaccination with Parents and Patients

Helen Bedford and Helen Donovan

6.1 Introduction

As is often observed, after clean water, vaccination is the most effective public health measure saving millions of lives and sparing people from illness and from serious complications. It therefore can be difficult to understand why people would question the value of vaccination. In the UK, vaccine programmes have successfully reduced the number of cases of many once common infectious diseases. For example, in 1967, the year before the introduction of the single measles vaccine, there were 460,407 notifications of measles and 99 deaths in England and Wales (UKHSA 2024a), and 50 years later in 2017, there were fewer than 2000 notifications with only 283 confirmed as measles (UKHSA 2023). These vaccination successes can result in a belief that vaccination is no longer necessary resulting in reduced vaccine uptake and an upsurge in cases as occurred in the UK in 2023/2024 (Bedford and Elliman, 2024).

6.2 What Is Vaccine Hesitancy?

Many factors contribute to low vaccine uptake (Chap. 12), including "vaccine hesitancy", defined by the World Health Organization (WHO) as "a delay in acceptance or refusal of vaccines despite availability of vaccination services" (World Health Organization 2014). The WHO emphasised the complexity of vaccine hesitancy with variation according to type of vaccine, location and time. Three influential factors (the "3Cs") were identified (see Fig. 6.1):

H. Bedford (✉)
Great Ormond Street Institute of Child Health, University College London, London, UK
e-mail: h.bedford@ucl.ac.uk

H. Donovan
Specialist in Immunisation and Vaccination, Independent Nurse Consultant, London, UK

© Springer Nature Switzerland AG 2025
H. Donovan, H. Bedford (eds.), *Safe Vaccine Administration*,
https://doi.org/10.1007/978-3-031-92498-9_6

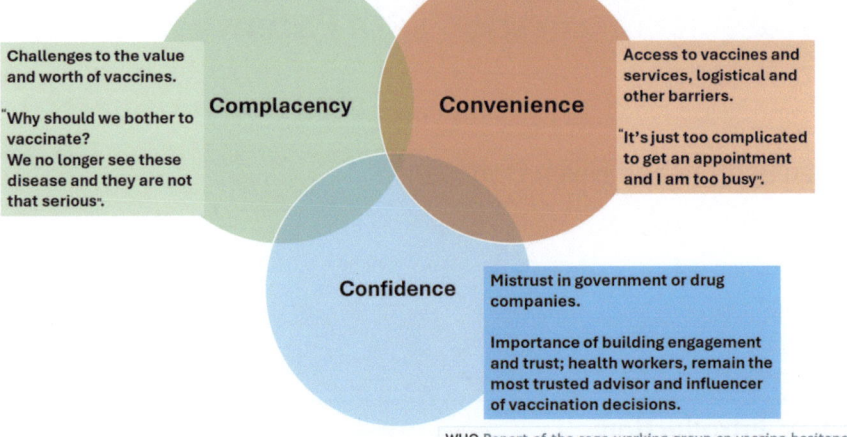

Fig. 6.1 The complexity of vaccine hesitancy. *Developed by the authors based on the WHO Report of the sage working group on vaccine hesitancy*

- *Complacency:* where vaccination is not considered necessary due to low disease risk.
- *Confidence:* this includes having trust in the vaccines themselves and their safety and efficacy, the pharmaceutical companies developing and marketing them, the health system and personnel delivering them and governments and policymakers making decisions about vaccination programmes.
- *Convenience:* ease of access to vaccination services and to vaccine information. Both physically accessing and understanding it.

None of these influences are independent. For example, an individual who has concerns about vaccines or considers them to be unnecessary may also experience challenges making a convenient appointment; this difficulty may reinforce their complacency. The original WHO definition was initially developed to include issues around difficulties accessing vaccination (Bedford et al. 2018); however, vaccine hesitancy has increasingly come to be used primarily to refer to parents/patients with doubts or concerns about vaccination which may prevent or delay them from being vaccinated.

While this distinction may seem very academic for those involved in providing vaccine programmes, an agreed definition is important for accurate measurement; vaccine hesitancy is often described as being on the increase. In addition, the issues preventing uptake need to be understood to plan appropriate services and to ensure provision of more effective, relevant vaccine conversations with the public. More recently, vaccine hesitancy has been redefined as "… a motivational state of being conflicted about, or opposed to, getting vaccinated; this includes intentions and willingness" (World Health Organization 2022), thus separating it from the resultant behaviour which may depend on external factors such as how services are provided, over which parents and patients may have little influence.

In the UK, the degree of hesitancy toward childhood vaccines is unclear, but many more parents have questions and concerns than actually decline vaccines. As discussed in Chap. 12, surveys consistently show a high level of vaccine confidence in the routine childhood programme (Campbell et al. 2017, 2023; Sherman et al. 2023, Skirrow et al. 2024b) despite recent small declines (UKHSA 2024a, b).

6.3 Impact of COVID-19 Pandemic on Public Attitudes to Vaccination

During the pandemic, unprecedented attention was given to vaccination with the rapid development of safe and effective vaccines hailed as "one of science's greatest achievements" (Griffin 2024). A surge of information followed from different sources. This "infodemic" included misinformation causing mistrust and confusion about what information to believe (WHO 2025). Anti-vaccine groups in particular, previously a fringe movement focused mainly on childhood vaccination, capitalized on the universality of COVID, on fears of infection and objections to public health measures introduced to reduce transmission of infection and spread disinformation widely on social media about the origins and/or severity of COVID infection and perceived rapid vaccine development (Carpiano et al. 2023). This may also have resulted in increasing hesitancy toward established vaccines. While there is little evidence to suggest this has severely dented confidence in routine childhood vaccination in the UK, where once people may have automatically accepted vaccines, parents, particularly from minority ethnic groups, report having more questions about routine vaccination since the COVID-19 pandemic (Skirrow et al. 2024a). There is also evidence that younger parents may be less vaccine confident (Eagan et al. 2023).

6.4 The Value of Vaccine Conversations

It is understandable and should be expected that people have questions and concerns about vaccination, just as they would for any medical procedure. It is important therefore that healthcare professionals are equipped to respond effectively. However, an effective response does not just involve giving facts to fill a "knowledge gap" or correcting misinformation—the style of conversation is important to build trust and confidence. Communication is a key aspect of nursing care (Nursing and Midwifery Council 2024). Providing evidence-based information in a supportive and compassionate way is a fundamental nursing skill embracing both the art and the science of nursing. It is an art ensuring people can understand, engage with and trust information as well as being aware of its sound scientific basis; this is an important part of maintaining public trust in vaccination.

Vaccine conversations with health professionals have been shown to influence parents' decisions about vaccination with a recommendation to vaccinate from a health professional associated with vaccine acceptance (Smith et al., 2017). The UKHSA report that although most parents have decided to vaccinate before a discussion, a significant proportion decide to vaccinate as a result of the discussion (UKHSA 2024a, b). However, UK studies find that while most parents report receiving vaccine information from health professionals, with a high proportion reporting feeling more confident following such a discussion (UKHSA 2023), some feel they are not provided with answers to all their questions (Skirrow et al. 2024b). Importantly, the UKHSA reported that almost 40% of parents who had refused or delayed a vaccine felt they had not had enough information compared with 14% who had (Campbell et al. 2023).

Trust is a key influence on vaccine acceptance—in the safety and effectiveness of the product, in the health system as a whole and in the advice given. Most parents report trusting immunisation information provided by the NHS and by health professionals and wanting more opportunities to discuss their questions with a trusted health professional (Skirrow et al. 2024a, b).

Leaflets and online information are also valuable to reinforce vaccine conversations but should not replace a conversation with a health professional (Skirrow et al. 2024a, b). In the absence of information from health professionals, patients and parents turn to other sources of information, some of which may be unreliable, fuelling misinformation.

See Fig. 6.2 for a nurse having conversation with mother and baby and discussing the child's red book.

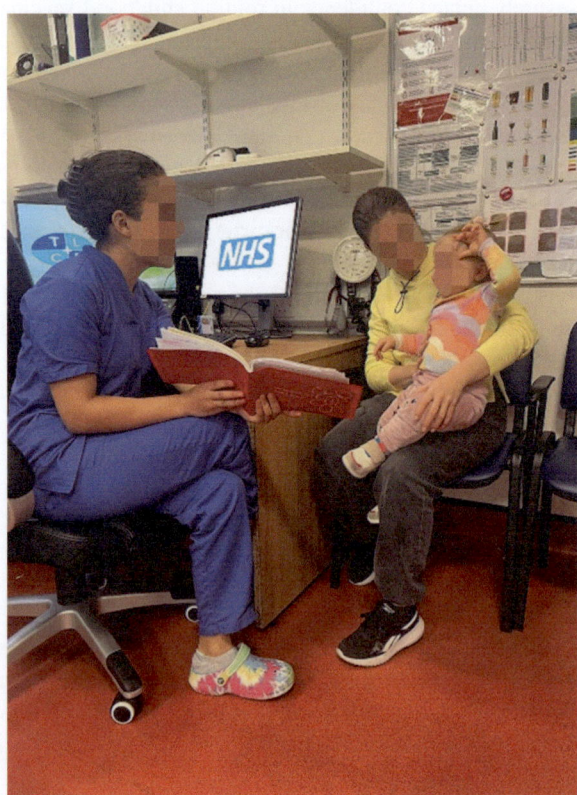

Fig. 6.2 Nurse discussing vaccines with mother and baby

6.5 Timing of Vaccine Information Provision

Parents express wanting more information about childhood vaccination during their pregnancy or soon after birth, and, while many parents do receive information before their baby's first vaccination appointment, many do not have a discussion until the appointment. This leaves an important gap for vaccine hesitant parents who, without the opportunity to discuss their questions in advance with a healthcare professional, may decide not to attend the appointment. Highlighting where to access reliable information early on for parents, e.g. during pregnancy or soon after birth, and advising them that healthcare professionals are available to discuss their questions and how they can get in touch to do this are important.

6.6 Frequently Asked Questions

Many questions about vaccination are predictable, with vaccine safety in particular a common concern. This means that health professionals can be prepared about specific issues with resources to hand to support their discussions. However, while it might be tempting to use prepared answers to these questions, this can be limiting as it is important to listen to the specific concern and particular nuance or context to their question to provide a tailored response. Nor it is recommended to simply give more and more facts—people may be more receptive to a more conversational style of communication rather than a lecture aimed at filling a knowledge gap (Bedford and Elliman 2024).

The following are some frequently asked questions:

- Are vaccines safe?
- The diseases have disappeared, so why still vaccinate?
- Why do we need to immunise babies at such a young age?
- I am breastfeeding—won't that protect my baby against these infections?
- What are the ingredients in vaccines and will they cause harm?
- Isn't "natural immunity" better?
- I use homeopathy and do not want to have conventional vaccines.
- Don't all these vaccines overload the immune system?
- I am worried that MMR vaccine causes autism.

6.7 Principles of Discussing Vaccination with Parents and Patients

There are many published guidelines and articles about vaccination communication/conversations (e.g. Leask et al. 2012; Bedford and Elliman 2020; World Health Organization 2021; Whitehead et al. 2023; Opel 2023; O'Leary 2025; Jitsuvax 2025); despite differences in the detail, the principles are similar. This involves using the principles of motivational interviewing and a guiding style (Leask et al., 2012).

In this chapter, these principles will be discussed using the example of a child who is delayed having their MMR vaccine because of parental fears about the safety of the vaccine; this is not intended as a comprehensive guide to vaccine conversations which are inevitably complex. The focus will be on the *style* of communication rather than the facts about the vaccine which can be found elsewhere, e.g. Oxford Vaccine Group (Appendix 1).

> **Case Study**
> A 5-year-old child, Jay, attends the GP for his asthma. On reviewing the child's records, it appears he has all his childhood vaccines with the exception of MMR vaccine. On discussion, it emerges that his parents have been reluctant to accept the MMR vaccine because they have read it causes autism.

6.8 Conversation Fundamentals

- **Ask permission to discuss.**
- **Listen to and elicit concerns.**
- **Show empathy and understanding.**

As Jay is 5 and has a medical condition, it is likely his parents have been asked about MMR several times before, and so they may feel defensive if the subject is broached again. Acknowledging that it is very positive that they have accepted all the other vaccines and asking their permission to discuss the issue may make them feel more in control.

Asking open questions rather than questions which may elicit only yes/no answers is more likely to encourage discussion and show a willingness to listen. For example, "What are your questions?" invites questions and validates that it is okay to have them, in contrast with "Do you have any questions?"

In view of the wealth of information readily available online and via social media, some of which is unreliable, it is not surprising for parents to have concerns about vaccination. Expressing empathy and understanding about these concerns may help gain a parent's trust and confidence. For example:

"I see that Jay has had all his vaccines except MMR. It is not surprising with all the information around that you might be worried about this vaccine, what are your questions and concerns?"

A vital part of the discussion is to listen to parents'/patients' concerns and avoid making assumptions about the reasons a vaccine has been delayed or declined. This facilitates a response tailored to their specific concerns, which is likely to be more impactful. It may also be useful to enquire if the parents have read or heard any information and the source of that—this helps you to judge if it is reliable and how you may need to respond. It is also important to be respectful of concerns and questions and not to dismiss them without discussion. Although some concerns can occasionally appear extreme, to the parents they are sufficiently concerning to have caused them to delay vaccination and they need to be responded to appropriately.

6.9 Correcting/Debunking Misinformation

Evidence suggests that correcting misinformation or "debunking" too vigorously can sometimes backfire, by reinforcing a belief. However, there is also evidence that anticipating the misinformation and "getting it out of the way" early on in the discussion can be effective (Whitehead et al. 2023). For example, making the statement:

"There is strong evidence from multiple studies showing no link between MMR vaccine and autism. On the other hand the original paper suggesting a link has been widely dis-credited".

This statement may of course need to be elaborated on depending on the parent's response.

Guidance (Jitsuvax 2025) suggests that even when a belief is expressed that is not scientifically accurate, it may be valuable to acknowledge a partial truth. For example, a common concern is that multiple or combination vaccines overload the immune system:

"It does seem like a lot of vaccines all at once, doesn't it? But compared with what we are all exposed to every day, lots of bacteria, viruses and other foreign material, in fact right from birth, the amount contained in vaccines is minimal. Nowadays vaccines are highly refined and give a controlled dose of the substance needed to stimulate a child's immune system, so they develop protection without the risks of having a full blown disease. Vaccines actually strengthen the immune system and are much less likely to cause serious problems than the diseases".

6.10 Giving Information About the Diseases and the Vaccines

The success of vaccination programmes means that fewer people experience the diseases. Despite outbreaks of measles and whooping cough, most parents have no experience of looking after a very sick child, and in this context, it can be challenging conveying the severity and consequence of vaccine preventable diseases; in the absence of disease, the risks of vaccination may seem greater. Using comparators familiar to parents may be helpful such as comparing the rates of severe consequences of measles with the rates of serious side effects of MMR vaccine in a 1000 pupil school. Sharing your professional experiences of diseases, of vaccinating or of personal vaccine decisions can also be helpful (if you are willing to share) demonstrating that you follow your own advice.

It is always important to advise parents about the common, minor side effects of the vaccine as well as rare, serious ones and how to manage them. This is particularly important for MMR vaccine due to the delayed onset of side effects such as fever and appearance of the side effects of the three vaccine components at different times (Vaccine Knowledge Project; Bedford and Elliman 2020). A hesitant parent who decides to have their child vaccinated may become very concerned if not prepared, for example, if they develop a fever a week or later following vaccination. Following the first primary vaccines, what may seem like mild side effects to a health professional may be perceived as serious to a parent whose 8-week-old baby is experiencing their first fever.

6.11 Unhelpful Strategies

Being aware of strategies that are less helpful to gain confidence and trust is also important. For example, using a directive or even argumentative approach, making comments such as "this is what you should do", suggesting the parents do not care about their child's welfare, belittling, dismissing or being disrespectful of questions and concerns and suggesting that you are the expert and therefore know best may lead to dissatisfaction with the conversation and the experience as a whole resulting in no further engagement by the parents.

6.12 Leaving the Door Open

If, following the discussion, the parent is still not ready to make a vaccine decision, it is important that the door is left open for further discussion. Ideally, it should be made clear that while you strongly recommend vaccination, it is the parent's decision (this may help parents feel more in control), and an opportunity for further discussion is always available, advising that although timely vaccination is preferable, it is never too late to have most vaccines.

6.13 Conclusion

In this chapter, some principles that can contribute to an effective vaccine conversation with parents and patients have been discussed. Many resources are available to support such conversations (Appendix 1). Effective vaccine conversations need skill and often require time, which can be a challenge in busy primary care settings, but it is time spent well as they are invaluable in supporting vaccine decision-making.

References

Bedford H. Elliman D. Measles rates are rising again. BMJ 2024; 382: q259
Bedford, H., Attwell, K., Danchin, M., Marshall, H., Corben, P. and Leask, J., 2018. Vaccine hesitancy, refusal and access barriers: The need for clarity in terminology. Vaccine, 36(44), pp.6556-6558.
Bedford, H.E. and Elliman, D.A., 2020. Fifteen-minute consultation: Vaccine-hesitant parents. Archives of Disease in Childhood-Education and Practice, 105(4), pp.194–199.
Campbell, H., Edwards, A., Letley, L., Bedford, H., Ramsay, M. and Yarwood, J., 2017. Changing attitudes to childhood immunisation in English parents. Vaccine, 35(22), pp.2979–2985.
Campbell, H., Paterson, P., Letley, L., Saliba, V., Mounier-Jack, S. and Yarwood, J., 2023. Vaccination, information and parental confidence in the digital age in England. *Vaccine: X, 14*, p.100345.
Carpiano, R.M., Callaghan, T., DiResta, R., Brewer, N.T., Clinton, C., Galvani, A.P., Lakshmanan, R., Parmet, W.E., Omer, S.B., Buttenheim, A.M. and Benjamin, R.M., 2023. Confronting the evolution and expansion of anti-vaccine activism in the USA in the COVID-19 era. The Lancet, 401(10380), pp.967–970.
Eagan, R.L., Larson, H.J. and de Figueiredo, A., 2023. Recent trends in vaccine coverage and confidence: a cause for concern. *Human Vaccines & Immunotherapeutics, 19*(2), p.2237374.
Griffin P. 2024 One of science's greatest achievements: how the rapid development of COVID vaccines prepares us for future pandemics. The Conversation, October 7th https://theconversation.com/one-of-sciences-greatest-achievements-how-the-rapid-development-of-covid-vaccines-prepares-us-for-future-pandemics-228787
Leask, J., Kinnersley, P., Jackson, C., Cheater, F., Bedford, H. and Rowles, G., 2012. Communicating with parents about vaccination: a framework for health professionals. BMC pediatrics, 12, pp.1–11.
Nursing and Midwifery Council (2024) The Code: Professional standards of practice and behaviour for nurses, midwives and nursing associates - The Nursing and Midwifery Council
O'Leary S. 2025. Strategies for Communicating With Parents About Vaccines JAMA. 2025; 333(24):2197–2198. https://doi.org/10.1001/jama.2025.4882
Opel, D.J., 2023. Clinician communication to address vaccine hesitancy. Pediatric Clinics, 70(2), pp.309-319.
Sherman, S.M., Lingley-Heath, N., Lai, J., Sim, J. and Bedford, H., 2023. Parental acceptance of and preferences for administration of routine varicella vaccination in the UK: A study to inform policy. Vaccine, 41(8), pp.1438–1446.
Skirrow, H., Lewis, C., Haque, H., Choundary-Salter, L., Foley, K., Whittaker, E., Costelloe, C., Bedford, H. and Saxena, S., 2024a. The impact of the COVID-19 pandemic on UK parents' attitudes towards routine childhood vaccines: A mixed-methods study. Plos one, 19(8), p.e0306484.
Skirrow, H., Lewis, C., Haque, H., Choudary-Salter, L., Foley, K., Whittaker, E., Costelloe, C., Bedford, H. and Saxena, S., 2024b. 'Why did nobody ask us?': A mixed-methods co-produced study in the United Kingdom exploring why some children are unvaccinated or vaccinated late. Vaccine, 42(22), p.126172.
Smith, L.E., Amlôt, R., Weinman, J., Yiend, J. and Rubin, G.J., 2017. A systematic review of factors affecting vaccine uptake in young children. *Vaccine, 35*(45), pp.6059–6069.
The Jitsuvax Project 2025. Addressing vaccine misinformation with health workers. https://jitsuvax.info/
UKHSA 2024a. Measles notifications and deaths in England and Wales: 1940 to 2023. https://www.gov.uk/government/publications/measles-deaths-by-age-group-from-1980-to-2013-ons-data/measles-notifications-and-deaths-in-england-and-wales-1940-to-2013

UKHSA 2024b. Childhood vaccines: parental attitudes survey 2023 findings. https://www.gov.uk/government/publications/childhood-vaccines-parental-attitudes-survey-2023/childhood-vaccines-parental-attitudes-survey-2023-findings

UKHSA 2023. Confirmed cases of measles, mumps and rubella in England and Wales: 1996 to 2022. https://www.gov.uk/government/publications/measles-confirmed-cases/confirmed-cases-of-measles-mumps-and-rubella-in-england-and-wales-2012-to-2013

Whitehead, H.S., French, C.E., Caldwell, D.M., Letley, L. and Mounier-Jack, S., 2023. A systematic review of communication interventions for countering vaccine misinformation. Vaccine, 41(5), pp.1018–1034.

World Health Organization 2021. How to talk about vaccines. https://www.who.int/news-room/feature-stories/detail/how-to-talk-about-vaccines

World Health Organization. Report of the SAGE working Group on vaccine hesitancy; 2014. http://www.who.int/immunization/sage/meetings/2014/october/1_Report_WORKING_GROUP_vaccine_hesitancy_final.pdf.

World Health Organization. 2022. Understanding the behavioural and social drivers of vaccine uptake WHO position paper—May 2022. Weekly Epidemiological Record 2022; 20 (97): 209–224. https://iris.who.int/bitstream/handle/10665/354458/WER9720-eng-fre.pdf?sequence=1

WHO. 2025. Infodemic https://www.who.int/health-topics/infodemic#tab=tab_1

Principles and Practice of Consent in Relation to Vaccine Administration

7

Helen Donovan, Sarah Lang, David Green, and Chris Green

7.1 Introduction to Consent

Consent is defined by the legal dictionary (2015 online) as "permission for something to happen or agreement to do something". Before a vaccination can be administered, informed consent must be obtained, just as with any healthcare intervention.

Consent must be freely given without coercion, by someone who is appropriately informed and who has the capacity and understanding to make the decision.

Obtaining consent is a process between the individual providing the care and the individual or their representative. This may be from the parent or guardian, for a child too young to give informed consent or where an adult lacks capacity to consent themselves, as a "best interest decision" for the treatment, in consultation with the individual's representative.

In order to give consent for a vaccine, the person needs to have the appropriate information about the vaccine being offered and an opportunity to consider and discuss it, as necessary. Robust consent processes support the delivery of quality and timely vaccination programmes and encourage trust within it.

H. Donovan (✉)
Specialist in Immunisation and Vaccination, Independent Nurse Consultant, London, UK

S. Lang · C. Green
London, UK

D. Green
Immunisation programmes: Design, Implementation and Clinical Guidance Division, UK Health Security Agency, London, UK

7.2 Legal Position and Policy

Consent is a key aspect of any healthcare intervention and a fundamental legal and ethical principle which all vaccinators need to be knowledgeable about as set out in the National Minimum Standards and Core Curriculum for Vaccination Training UKHSA (2025). The process and principles for consent in a vaccination context are set out in Chap. 2 in the "Green Book" and also the RCN consent guide 2022 which has separate sections for the principles for Consent in England and Wales, Consent in Northern Ireland and Consent in Scotland.

While the broad principles of the law of consent are the same in all parts of the UK, there are legislative differences between countries. Links to further country specific legislation/guidance are provided in Box 7.1.

> **Box 7.1 Country Specific Legislation**
> England and Wales: Mental Capacity Act 2005;
> Scotland: Adults with Incapacity (Scotland) Act 2000, Mental Health (Care and Treatment) (Scotland) Act 2003 Mental Health (Scotland) Act 2015) Age of legal capacity (Scotland) Act 1991)
> Northern Ireland: Mental Health (Northern Ireland) Order 1986, Mental Capacity Act (Northern Ireland) 2016

7.3 Basic Principles of Consent

In England, Wales and Northern Ireland, anyone under 18 is a "child". In Scotland, a "child" is under the age of 16 and older teenagers are considered "adults". Otherwise, the same principles apply throughout the UK.

Adults
- An adult with capacity (see below; can the individual give consent?) must freely consent, without coercion, before treatment is given.
- Consent is only valid if the patient has sufficient information about the benefits and risks of treatment.
- Consent may be communicated verbally or in writing or may be inferred from the patient's actions (e.g. if a patient reads the information leaflet and then silently offers her arm for injection, this might constitute a valid consent).
- Consent may be withdrawn at any time before the treatment has been given.
- If the adult lacks capacity, then the treatment may be given if it is the best interests of the patient, in accordance with the relevant mental capacity regulations and guidance.

Children

- Adults with parental responsibility may give consent on behalf of their children.
- In England, Wales and Northern Ireland, children with capacity aged 16 or 17 may consent to their own treatment, whether their parents give consent or not (in Scotland, this issue does not arise since 16- and 17-year-olds are considered adults).
- A child under the age of 16 who is capable of understanding the nature and possible consequences of the treatment may give a valid consent (this is known as "Gillick competence").
- If there is dispute between parents, the family court may need to decide whether or not the treatment is given.
- Parental refusal can only be overridden in an emergency—if the treatment is *immediately* necessary and in the best interests of the child, it may lawfully be given, even if the parents do not consent. This situation is highly unlikely with vaccination (a possible example might be for a child, bitten by a rabid dog—the nurse might proceed with an urgent rabies vaccine even if the parents do not consent).
- Key issues that can arise around this will be discussed later in the chapter.

7.4 Consent Process: Information and Dialogue

Consent, as described earlier, is a legal necessity, but the process also presents an opportunity for vaccinators to engage with patients/parents/carers building positive relationships and consolidating trust.

There is no legal requirement for consent to vaccination to be in writing, and a signature on a consent form is not necessary. In practice, most vaccines are administered following verbal consent which is obtained through a consultation with the individual or their representative. A consent form is often used in school-based vaccine programmes or in occupational health settings. The consent forms, whether paper or electronic, capture health information and individual or parental consent of students or individuals vaccinated in single vaccine sessions.

Any vaccinators using consent forms outside of these settings should consider their necessity and reflect if they could be introducing an unnecessary barrier to vaccination. The process of consent should focus on being voluntary and informed and a signature on a consent form alone is not conclusive proof that a valid consent has been given.

Consent may also be implied rather than expressed verbally or in writing. This would mean that the individual's actions and the circumstances around these would indicate that they are consenting. Nurses do need, however, to make sure they are confident the person has had the information they need.

7.5 Practice Issue: Informed Consent Vs Implied Consent

Consider practice scenario 1 in Box 7.2:

> **Box 7.2 Practice Issue Scenario 1**
> 1. **A mother brings in her child for the pre-school vaccines with her invitation for the vaccine to be given.**
>   She sits down and holds the child ready for their vaccines and just wants to get on with it. Is this consent by implication?
>   How does this align with the principles discussed so far?
>
> *All individuals should be offered standard information, and it is best practice for the vaccinator to ensure that the individual has had information and that they understand this.*

7.6 Informed Consent

Whether the consent process is through a face to face or telephone consultation, or utilising a consent form, it should be "informed". Before giving consent, the patient should be made aware of the benefits and risks of the treatment (including rare and common side effects and what to do if they occur) and of the consequences of them not receiving the treatment See Box 7.3. Skilled vaccinators must be able to provide tailored, appropriate and accurate information for everyone they are obtaining consent from. This principle informs best practice that information is provided to an individual, either verbally if consulting face to face or having a follow-up phone call or in writing in the form of a leaflet or information on the consent form, for school-based programmes.

> **Box 7.3 Standard Information to Include in the Consent Process**
> - The vaccine/s to be given
> - The disease(s) the vaccine is helping to prevent
> - The benefits and risk of vaccination vs. the risks of disease(s)
> - Possible side effects of the vaccine and how to manage these
> - Any follow-up recommended or additional doses of vaccine
> - How data will be used and stored

The range and depth of information that individuals will need in order to give consent can vary. Some require very little information while others have many questions. Vaccinators should utilise good communication skills including expressing empathy and active listening to elicit concerns and meet the information needs of each individual.

The legal requirement is to inform the patient of any "material risks". A risk is "material" if a reasonable person in the patient's position would be likely to attach significance to the risk or if the nurse should reasonably be aware that this particular patient will attach significance to the risk. Consider practice scenarios 2, 3 and 4 in Box 7.4:

> **Box 7.4 Practice Issues Scenarios 2–4—"Material Risk"—How Much Information Should You Give About Risks?**
> 2. Paul is a 17-year-old boy with haemophilia, attending for a hepatitis B vaccine. The risks of a haematoma at the injection site are very low in the general population, but significant in haemophiliacs.
>   *This is therefore a reasonable risk for Paul to consider and it should be discussed with him.*
> 3. Joanna is a 30-year-old businesswoman. She is a member of an "anti-vax" group. She needs to travel to Sierra Leone on business and finds out that she will not be allowed to enter the country without proof of yellow fever vaccination. Reluctantly, she makes enquiries at her GP surgery.
>   *Travel vaccines are discussed in Chap. 2 and the resources for yellow fever and the associated risks included. While the risks to Joanna are extremely low, she is known to be very suspicious of vaccines and is likely to find them significant. In this situation, it is, therefore, necessary to discuss the risks with her in detail so that she can make a fully informed decision whether to go ahead with the vaccination.*
> 4. Hilary, age 21, is a healthcare worker and part-time model, who has an occupational health appointment for a BCG vaccination. The vaccination might leave a small scar at the injection site.
>   *While the scar is usually unobtrusive, Hilary is likely to consider it significant and it should be discussed with her.*

Assessing understanding of the information provided is an important part of safe practice.

For example, ensure that a contraindication is not missed or that language or capacity issues have not been identified.

The resources below can be used to both convey information and check understanding. For some vaccines, there are checklists available to work through with a patient prior to vaccination—best practice would include showing these to the patient to view while verbalizing to minimise risks of misunderstanding.

7.7 Information Resources

There is a wide range of vaccine information available, and this can be provided in written as well as verbal formats. Written information can include leaflets, weblinks or utilising some of the other tools in the clinical setting. Information should be tailored to the individual or particular population groups. See the resources section of this book as well as Chap. 6 "Vaccine Conversations" and Chap. 12 "Maximising Uptake" for more information.

Consideration must be given to potential barriers to obtaining consent, such as language and literacy issues or particular concerns about vaccines within a community. These must be promptly identified and addressed. Health inequalities exist, and unvaccinated individuals are often in vulnerable groups or within under vaccinated demographic populations—this can in turn sustain disease transmission and further exacerbate health inequalities (see Box 7.5).

> **Box 7.5 Information Giving Summary**
> - For many patients, the consent process is straightforward, the information is understood and the consent is given.
> - For a small number of patients, the process maybe more complex before consent can be obtained, and the vaccine given.
> - Providing information tailored to individuals is an important part of the consent process.
> - Good communication supports the development of positive relationships between patients and vaccinators which in turn may support the development of trust—a cornerstone of vaccine confidence.

7.8 Resources in Other Languages

Many of the resources are available in a range of languages and in different formats like video. Where translations aren't available, google translate offers the facility to translate whole webpages or specific documents—simply open Google Translate and copy the text or webpage address to translate. Local NHS services may also have resources in other languages and for groups with low literacy levels videos or sound recordings. See Box 7.6 for a summary.

7.9 Easy Read Leaflets

These are available for some vaccine programmes, for example, influenza and COVID-19 vaccines, to support the use with individuals with learning disabilities.

7.10 Language Interpretation

The Migrant Health Guide (Migrant health guide—GOV.UK (www.gov.uk) (OHID 2025) from the Office for Health Improvement and Disparities further provides advice and guidance on the health needs of migrant patients including language interpretation. The webpage has links to guidelines and resources to support clinical practice. Many of the leaflets and resources for the UK routine programme are available in many languages and available to order free of charge for vaccinators.

7.11 Literacy Issues

Consider any groups in whom literacy could be an issue—are there other media available that could be used to communicate key health messages, for example, translated audio recordings/videos or pictures?

7.12 Supporting the Consent Process

The consent process as described above is dependent on several factors which include skilled vaccinators, time afforded within consultations to allow for consent conversations and motivation to work within best practice to deliver a successful vaccination programme. Any barriers, real or potential, should be identified and promptly addressed.

7.13 Gaining Consent: Practice Based Issues

This section will concentrate on some of the issues that may arise when seeking consent for vaccines in practice.

7.14 Can the Individual Provide Consent? Do They Have the Capacity?

Vaccinators must ensure that the individual they are seeking consent from either has the capacity or legal authority to do so.

Adults: Adults aged 18 years and over (16 or over in Scotland) are assumed to have capacity to consent for their own treatment unless and until it is established that they do not have capacity. For example, nurses should not assume that an adult patient with a learning disability lacks capacity but should ask questions. A patient who shows an understanding of the benefits and risks of the vaccination has capacity, regardless of any learning disability. If a patient with capacity refuses vaccination, then that refusal must be respected, however unwise it may appear to the vaccinator.

If the patient lacks capacity, then the nurse may administer the vaccine if it is in the best interests of the patient. For example, a person with a learning disability has severe asthma but lacks capacity to consent to the influenza vaccine. If the nurse assesses that vaccination will be in the patient's best interests, they may lawfully administer the vaccine following a discussion with the patient's representative and in accordance with the relevant mental capacity regulations and guidance.

The legislation referenced in this chapter is specific to the geographical region of the UK in which vaccinators work. Local policies should be in place which incorporate the relevant legislation and provide a clear pathway for the vaccinator to follow. Clear local policies can facilitate vaccine provision and support vaccinators to work within legal boundaries. Ensuring staff have time to complete this work is essential, and the importance of obtaining consent should not be overlooked during periods of high-volume vaccine delivery such as during flu clinics. The principles of consent remain.

Children: Young people aged 16 and 17 years are legally considered adults in Scotland. In the remainder of the UK, they are presumed in law to be able to consent to medical treatment and as for adults should be assumed to have that capacity.

For the under 16s, consent will usually be obtained from someone who has parental responsibility for the child unless the vaccinator is confident the young person has sufficient understanding to consent for themselves. In vaccination practice, this is usually described as Gillick competence.

The assessment of a child for Gillick competence is about the child having sufficient understanding and ability to comprehend the information in order to make a decision—this will vary greatly between children of similar ages and therefore is always an individual assessment—there is no lower age. Children with any level of understanding should be included in consent discussions when appropriate—the principle of Gillick competence supports the vaccination of young persons to consent for themselves (Care Quality Commission CQC 2022, NSPCC 2022).

Gillick competence assessments are a regular part of school-based vaccine programmes working with young adolescents. They support timely delivery of vaccines to individuals who may otherwise miss out due to lack of returned consent forms or where young people are keen to have vaccines but parents are unwilling to consent. Consider scenario 5 in Box 7.6:

Box 7.6 Practice Issue Scenario 5

5. **A 14- year- old comes to a school vaccine session and requests a HPV vaccine but informs you that their parents don't want them to have it.**

    The vaccinator accesses the consent form and can see that the parent has declined the vaccine.

    Potential barrier for vaccinator: fear of repercussions from the parents, giving a vaccine against parental wishes

    However, if this 14-year-old is turned away, they get no benefit from the early protection from HPV

    What steps should be taken?

(continued)

Box 7.6 (continued)

The same principles of consent apply here—that the consent must be informed, voluntary and by someone with the capacity for consent.

This can only happen through a dialogue with the 14 year old to assess if they have sufficient intelligence and understanding of the HPV vaccine including side effects etc.

It is also important to consider the parents and to see if working with them can be facilitated. However, it is not legally necessary to contact the parents and fear of angry parents should not be a barrier to a 14 year old receiving a vaccine they are entitled to.

If a young person is deemed to be Gillick Competent and they consent to vaccination that decision is binding.

Withholding vaccines without an indication to do so is an act of omission, and healthcare professionals are responsible for decisions not to give, in the same way as for giving a treatment. Accurate documentation is essential to record all steps that were taken. Organisations may have additional governance systems in place that empower vaccinators to support these young people. Scottish legislation (Age of Legal Capacity (Scotland) Act 1991) should be reviewed for those working under its jurisdiction.

Children under 16 years who are not Gillick competent: Require consent from someone with parental responsibility. Individuals with parental responsibility are defined legally within each part of the UK and summarised in the Department of Health and Social Care "Parental Rights and Responsibilities" (DHSC – on line 2023).

Vaccinators should work closely with families to be clear who has attended for vaccines with the infant/child and if they have parental responsibility and if they don't then to establish if the person attending has been given permission to provide consent.

The consent of one person with parental responsibility is all that is necessary. For example, if one parent brings her baby in for vaccination, the nurse need not enquire whether or not the other parent consents. However, if the nurse becomes aware that the other parent objects to the vaccination, they not proceed until the dispute has been resolved, if necessary, by an order of the family court. Consider scenarios 6 and 7 in Box 7.7 and what steps the vaccinator needs to take to ensure they have obtained consent (DH 2009). If the young person themselves is considered Gillick competent, they can consent and the vaccination can proceed despite any disagreement between the parents Green book chapter 2 (UKHSA 2024).

Box 7.7 Practice Scenario 6 and 7

6. **Baby A's parents are invited by letter to bring Baby A to the clinic for an MMR vaccine. An information sheet about the vaccine is enclosed with the letter. Baby A is brought into the clinic by her child minder, who says that Baby A's mother asked her to "bring the baby in for her vaccination".**

   Here, the mother has received all the relevant information in advance and then asked the child minder to "bring the baby in for her vaccination". Therefore, the mother has consented in advance to the vaccines.

   Provided that there is no reason to doubt the word of the child minder, the nurse may lawfully administer the vaccine.

7. **Baby B is brought into the same clinic by his grandmother, who tells the nurse that Baby B's parents asked her to "let him have the injection provided it is safe"'.**

   Under Section 2(9) of the Children Act 1989, parents are entitled to delegate decisions on the medical treatment of their children to other persons.

   In this case, the parents have delegated the decision to the grandmother.
   The nurse should explain the benefits and potential risks. If the grandmother then consents, the nurse may lawfully administer the vaccine.

In both these scenarios, the nurse should exercise reasonable judgement and caution. If in doubt about the parents' intentions, they should try to clarify these, e.g. by telephoning a parent. If either infant's records include a note that the parents are hostile to vaccination, it might be best to defer the treatment until the parents can attend and engage in a full discussion themselves.

The person with parental responsibility does not necessarily need to be present at the time the immunisation is given.

Barriers to vaccination such as insisting on letters from parents should generally be avoided, and if vaccinators are unsure about consent issues and children, then Chap. 2 of the Green Book should be used and referred to, which comprehensively sets out policy on this. When consent is given by a person other than the individual, it should be clearly documented in the medical record.

7.15 Conclusion

All vaccinators should be fully trained and remain up to date on consent law, principles and policy that are applicable to the country and clinical setting in which they practice. Adherence to these supports safe and legal practice but also ensures that patients or parents accessing vaccination services are being well cared for. Good communication and care around issues such as consent can foster trust which is a key aspect of a successful vaccination programme.

References

Care Quality Commission CQC (2022) Gillick competency and Fraser guidelines. https://www.cqc.org.uk/guidance-providers/gps/gp-mythbusters/gp-mythbuster-8-gillick-competency-fraser-guidelines (Accessed January 2023)

DH (2009) Department of Health. Reference guide to consent for examination or treatment. Second edition 2009 https://assets.publishing.service.gov.uk/government/uploads/system/uploads/attachment_data/file/138296/dh_103653__1_.pdf. [Accessed January 2023]

DHSC – on line Department of Health and social care 'Parental Rights and responsibilities' Parental rights and responsibilities: Who has parental responsibility - GOV.UK (www.gov.uk) [Accessed January 2023]

Legal dictionary Informed Consent Informed Consent (2015 online)- Definition, Examples, Cases, Processes (legaldictionary.net) [Accessed January 2023]

NSPCC (2022) Gillick competency and Fraser guidelines. https://learning.nspcc.org.uk/child-protection-system/gillick-competence-fraser-guidelines [Accessed January 2023]

OHID Office for Health Improvement and Disparities (2025) Migrant Health Guide Migrant health guide - GOV.UK (www.gov.uk) [Accessed May 2025]

UKHSA (2024). Consent, chapter 2 in: Immunisation against Infectious Diseases. Editor Ramsay M. 2023. Accessed May 2025 https://www.gov.uk/government/publications/consent-the-green-book-chapter-2

UKHSA (2025). National Minimum Standards and Core Curriculum for Vaccination Training https://www.gov.uk/government/publications/national-minimum-standards-and-core-curriculum-for-immunisation-training-for-registered-healthcare-practitioners

Authorisation of Medicines: In Relation to Vaccines

8

David Green, Helen Donovan, Jo Jenkins, and William Malcolm

8.1 Introduction

The administration of all medicines, including vaccines, is regulated through the Medicines and Healthcare Products Regulatory Agency (MHRA), operating with a statutory framework set by the UK Government Department of Health and Social Care (DHSC). The legislation applies across the UK, and it includes authorisation and licensing of all medicines.

The Medicines Act first came into legislation in 1968 (Medicines Act Legislation 1968), following concerns about the use of the drug thalidomide in pregnancy and the resulting foetal damage. It was introduced to regulate the pharmaceutical industry and the supply of medicines to the public. Since 1968, there have been a number of amendments to the legislation. The current medicines legislation relating to the supply and administration of prescription only medicines is in the Human Medicines Regulations 2012 (HMR 2012) and subsequent Statutory Instruments providing amendment to the Regulations—these cover the supply and administration of all medicinal products.

Most clinical care involving supplying and/or administering medicines should be undertaken on an individual, patient-specific basis (i.e. the medicine is prescribed for an individual by a prescriber). Obtaining a signed prescription for each vaccine to be given in a busy clinic is not practical and in the past was a barrier for nurses

---

D. Green (✉)
Immunisation Programmes Division, UK Health Security Agency, London, UK
e-mail: david.green@ukhsa.gov.uk

H. Donovan
Specialist in Immunisation and Vaccination, Independent Nurse Consultant, London, UK

J. Jenkins
Director Medicines Governance, Medicines Use and Safety, Specialist Pharmacy Services, England, UK

W. Malcolm (Retired)
Pharmaceutical Adviser NHS National Services, Scotland, UK

© Springer Nature Switzerland AG 2025
H. Donovan, H. Bedford (eds.), *Safe Vaccine Administration*,
https://doi.org/10.1007/978-3-031-92498-9_8

taking on the role of vaccination (Nursing Standard 1989). There are now clear, legal mechanisms to allow for the safe supply and/or administration of medicines in specific situations by specified registered healthcare professionals without the need for a prescription. This has enabled vaccine clinics and vaccine administration to become increasingly led by non-prescribers, particularly registered nurses and pharmacists. The UKHSA Quality criteria for an effective Immunisation programme, states that vaccines need to be given within the regulatory framework for medicines administration (UKHSA 2025), this chapter describes what these are.

8.2 Legal Administration of Medicines

Medicines are authorised for use and marketing in the UK by the MHRA, based on the information submitted by the manufacturer. The detail of the authorisation is available from the MHRA in the Public Assessment Report (PAR)—how the medicine should be used is detailed in the Summary of Product Characteristics (SmPC) (see MHRA Marketing authorisations, variations and licensing guidance: detailed information).

When medicinal products are provided with a marketing authorisation, it will describe the terms under which the product may be prescribed, supplied and/or administered and is specific to both the medicine itself and the product's packaging (see Box 8.1). Any change to the product assembly, such as alteration to the packaging or quantity supplied, may alter the legal terms under which the product may be provided.

There may be occasions where it is in the best interests of patients to receive a licensed medicine outside the terms of the SmPC. This is known as "off-label" use of a medicine.

For example, the Green Book *Immunisation Against Infectious Diseases* (UKHSA (on line) n.d.) sometimes differs in its recommendations on the use of vaccines from that given in the manufacturer's SmPC. The recommendations in the Green Book and in the specific vaccine program, Guidance for Healthcare Professionals, are based on advice from the Joint Committee on Vaccination and Immunisation (JCVI) and based on the best available evidence. If this advice differs, the Green Book or National Guidance for Healthcare Practitioners resources should be followed.

8.3 Classification of Vaccines

> **Box 8.1 The Legislation Defines Three Categories of Medicine Which Determine Terms Under Which They May Be Supplied**
> - Prescription only medicines (POMs)—available under a valid prescription. This needs to be from an appropriate practitioner: a registered medical practitioner, dentist or an independent nonmedical prescriber (referred to here as the prescriber)

(continued)

> **Box 8.1** (continued)
> - Pharmacy medicines (P)—may be sold or supplied without a prescription but can only be sold or supplied from a registered pharmacy under the supervision of a pharmacist
> - General sales list (GSL) medicines—can be bought from a wide range of retail outlets without a prescription or professional supervision.

All vaccines are classified as prescription only medicines (POMs) which means they need to have the appropriate legal authority to be supplied and/or administered to a patient.

8.4 Patient Specific Direction (PSD)/Prescription

A patient specific direction (PSD), which may also be referred to as a prescription in practice, is the traditional and preferred way that medicines are supplied and/or administered to a named individual. The PSD provides the instruction for the medicine to be supplied and/or administered after the prescriber has assessed the person on an individual basis.

This instruction is written and then signed by an authorised prescriber: a doctor, dentist or nonmedical prescriber. It can be for one individual at a time or several named individuals, for example, named persons attending for an influenza vaccine clinic, whom the prescriber has individually assessed as being suitable to receive the vaccine (see Box 8.2).

> **Box 8.2 Patient Specific Directions (PSDs)—Summary, in Vaccination Services**
> - A PSD provides a written instruction from a prescriber to another healthcare practitioner to legally authorise them to administer a vaccine directly to a named individual or several named individuals.
> - PSDs are individually tailored to the needs of an individual and should be considered preferable to a PGD, where they can be provided in a timely manner without compromising patient access to vaccination services.
> - The prescriber is responsible for the assessment of the individual(s) named and the PSD providing directions in writing detailing the medicines to be supplied or administered.
> - The prescriber can delegate the administration of a medicine they have prescribed to an appropriately trained and competent individual.
>
> See at the end of this chapter for more information and the Specialist Pharmacy Services (SPS) guidance on the use of PSDs.

8.5 Alternative Authorisation for Medicines Relevant to Vaccination

A PSD is not required if there is an exemption with a specific alternative authorisation, as identified in the legislation. The HMR (Human Medicines Regulations 2012) includes several lawful exemptions, commonly referred to as medicines mechanisms, which can be utilised to administer vaccines without the need for a PSD.

The provision of vaccination should be readily available so that individuals can receive vaccines easily and not have to wait for long periods of time for appointments. While it is best practice for any medicine or treatment to be provided on a named patient basis, this does not always result in easily accessible and timely vaccine administration; it is not always easy to predict who will be coming into the clinic, and obtaining a PSD either in advance or at the time of presentation may put unnecessary barriers in the way.

In practice, unless the person administering the vaccine is an independent prescriber, it has become common practice for supply and/or administration of vaccines in non-prescriber led services, such as nurse led clinics, pharmacy clinics or school-based vaccination sessions, that the authorisation is via a Patient Group Direction (PGD), an accepted tool for the supply and or giving of vaccines (Kenny 2013).

The Human Medicines (Coronavirus and Influenza) (Amendment) Regulations 2020 introduced, in response to the COVID-19 pandemic, a national protocol, which offered the advantage over PGDs in that they, for the administration of COVID and influenza vaccines, allow the separation of tasks within the vaccination process as detailed in the national protocol. In turn, this facilitated an expanded vaccination workforce necessary to provide a rapid and mass response during the COVID pandemic.

The various mechanisms identified in the legislation are summarised in Box 8.3, and this chapter goes on to provide further detail noting that legislation is under continual review—readers are advised to ensure they are aware of any changes to the legal mechanisms or workforces who can utilise them.

Box 8.3 Summary of Alternative Authorisation Mechanisms Relevant to Vaccination
- *Patient group direction (PGD)*
  Medicines may be supplied and/or administered in accordance with a PGD (Schedule 16 of HMR 2012 legislation). See below for more information on PGDs and the SPS guidance.
- *Written instruction*
  Medicines may be supplied and/or administered by certain registered practitioners in accordance with the written directions of a doctor during an occupational health scheme (Schedule 17 of HMR 2012 legislation). See below under written instruction.

(continued)

> **Box 8.3** (continued)
>
> - *Schedule 17 exemptions for midwives*
>   Under Schedule 17 of the HMR 2012, there are further exemptions to allow for specific professionals to administer and/or supply certain listed medicines as part of their professional practice without the need for a prescription, PSD or PGD. This includes midwives and appropriately supervised student midwives to administer the hepatitis B vaccination where indicated.
> - *National protocol*
>   Under the emergency legislative changes in the Human Medicines (Coronavirus and Influenza) (Amendment) Regulations 2020, a new regulation, 247A, allows for COVID-19 and influenza vaccine delivery under a protocol in specific circumstances. For further detail, see below.
> - *Emergency medicines*
>   Certain medicines can be administered by anyone in an emergency without the need for any legal authorisation. This includes adrenaline 1 in 1000 which can be administered in an emergency for the purpose of saving life (Schedule 19 of HMR 2012 legislation). See below under "Medicines That May Be Administered in Emergency".

8.6 Patient Group Directions (PGDs)

A patient group direction provides a legal framework for certain registered healthcare professionals, listed in the legislation, to supply and/or administer medicines without the need for them to be prescribed.

A PGD is a written direction for the supply or administration of medicine to individuals in a defined group, who may or may not be individually identified before presentation for treatment (see Box 8.4 for the key principles for PGDs).

> **Box 8.4 Key Practice Considerations for Using PGDs**
> - The use of a PGD should be reserved for situations where this offers advantage for clinical care without compromising patient safety.
> - PGDs are not appropriate for use in all settings or for all medicines—for further advice, see advice from the Specialist Pharmacy Services on when PGDs can be used.
> - Organisations should have governance processes in place to consider all options before a service is designed or commissioned using PGDs.
> - Before use of a PGD is authorised, the organisation must ensure that PGDs are appropriate and legal and that relevant governance arrangements are in place.
>
> SPS have a range of resources supporting PGD use available at https://www.sps.nhs.uk/home/guidance/patient-group-directions/.

8.7 Who Can Use a PGD

The legislation is specific on who can work under a PGD. Registered nurses (RNs) can use PGDs, but registered nursing associates are not included in the legislation, and neither are unregistered staff, such as healthcare support workers (HCSW). Where these staff are supporting vaccination clinics, they will need a PSD or to be working under a national protocol where this is applicable and available (see below for more detail).

The MHRA (2017) state that only fully competent, qualified, trained professionals can use PGDs for the supply and/or administration of vaccines; PGDs cannot be used as part of training. NICE guidance on PGDs (NICE 2017) recommends that a comprehensive and appropriate training programme be provided for all people involved in using PGDs with an assessment of competency used post-training. Additionally, the Nursing and Midwifery Council (NMC) Code states that nurses must be up to date with skills and knowledge and use the best available evidence (NMC 2022). Relevant training in immunisation and vaccination is a key requirement for use of vaccine PGDs.

PGDs are a useful tool to allow for vaccines to be administered to those who need them in a timely manner. The legislation is clear on how PGDs should be developed and used. PGDs must include specific information and have a clear governance process to support their use. Box 8.5 provides a summary of the good governance required for using PGDs.

Box 8.5 Summary for Good Governance on Using PGDs
- The healthcare professional authorised to use the PGD must be the one to undertake the complete episode of care. This includes clinical assessment of the individual, ensuring the person has given consent, the administering or supplying of the vaccine and completion of the records.
- A healthcare professional working under a PGD cannot delegate any part of the process to another person, whether this is a support worker, a student or another registered professional able to work under the PGD.
- Where a vaccine is not an injection, a PGD may be written to allow the healthcare professional to supply the vaccine to an individual, or their carer, for subsequent self-administration or administration by another person; an example of this in practice is the administration of the intranasal "flu vaccine".
- Good clinical governance must be in place to ensure all immunisers are appropriately trained with support and supervision available.

There are national PGD templates for all the vaccines recommended within the routine immunisation schedule for use in England: (United Kingdom Health Security Agency; UKHSA) PGD templates (https://www.gov.uk/government/collections/immunisation-patient-group-direction-pgd).

The UKHSA templates have been signed by a doctor, nurse and pharmacist, from the national immunisation team, who led their development. The templates must have organisational authorisation in accordance with Schedule 16 of HMR 2012 from the local/national commissioner or provider before they can be used, for example, the NHS trust or commissioning organisation. See the SPS implementation guidance (Implementation—SPS - Specialist Pharmacy Service—The first stop for professional medicines advice).

These templates are also provided as a reference resource to NHS organisations in Wales (Public Health Wales Immunisation https://phw.nhs.wales/topics/immunisation-and-vaccines/) when developing their own PGDs.

There is a similar arrangement in Northern Ireland where the UKHSA templates are used as a reference and amended and authorised accordingly by a multidisciplinary team (HSCNI primary care PGD here).

In Scotland, national specimen PGDs for vaccines are produced by Public Health Scotland to assist NHS Boards to develop local PGDs (PHS Scotland PGD templates) (Publications—Public Health Scotland (search PGDs)).

8.8 Written Instructions

Under the legislation, occupational health services or schemes (OHS) may utilise an exemption from the restrictions that apply to the supply and administration of prescription only medicines (Schedule 17 HMR 2012).

An OHS is designed to help protect and promote workers' physical, mental and social health and well-being. Medicinal products can be supplied or administered during an occupational health service by a registered practitioner acting in accordance with the written and signed instruction of a doctor, commonly documented as a written instruction. A written instruction is not subject to the legislated framework of a PGD, and a written instruction is not interchangeable with a PGD. A written instruction template is available from the BMA document "The Occupational Physician" Appendix 6 (BMA 2019).

Apart from flu and coronavirus vaccines, a written instruction is an arrangement between a named registered nurse or group of named registered nurses and an authorising OHS doctor to allow for the supply and/or administration of a medicine for an occupational health purpose. No other healthcare professionals can work under an OHS written instruction.

Vaccines given in the course of an OHS should be undertaken using a written instruction or a PSD (SPS PGDs and Occupational Health Schemes) (Occupational Health Services—SPS—Specialist Pharmacy Service—The first stop for professional medicines advice).

Where influenza or coronavirus vaccines are given as part of an NHS or local authority (LA) OHS, including peer to peer vaccinations, the legislation allows for a wider group of healthcare professionals to work under these specific written instructions—this group of registered healthcare professional is termed "occupational health vaccinators" and includes registered midwives, pharmacists and nursing associates—for further detail, see Using written instructions in occupational health services—SPS—Specialist Pharmacy Service—The first stop for professional medicines advice.

To support the delivery of the influenza vaccine and peer to peer vaccination, there is a written instruction template specifically for influenza vaccine which can be adopted by organisations available at the link above (SPS 2024).

8.9 National Protocol

The national protocol option was introduced as part of the emergency legislative changes to the Human Medicines (Coronavirus and Influenza) (Amendment) Regulations 2020. The new regulation, 247A, allows for COVID-19 and influenza vaccine delivery under a national protocol in specific circumstances.

The national protocol allows the vaccination process to be separated into specific tasks or stages (consent and clinical assessment, preparation, administration and record-keeping). The national protocol details who can undertake each stage (i.e. listed registered healthcare professionals, unregistered healthcare professionals, etc.). Only registered healthcare professionals listed in the protocol are able to undertake the consent and clinical assessment stages; they may also undertake the other stages, or these may be subsequently undertaken by another healthcare professional, as detailed within the national protocol. This is in contrast to a PGD where the entire process has to be undertaken by a single registered healthcare professional working under the PGD.

This separation of stages of the vaccination process can improve workflow and increase the available workforce.

The legislation is due to expire in April 2026, as it stands it is not expected to be extended nor made permanent. As previously stated, vaccinators need to make sure they are aware of any changes to the legal mechanisms for vaccine supply and/or administration and to the workforces who can utilise them.

8.10 Schedule 17 Exemptions for Midwives

Schedule 17 of the HMR 2012 exemptions allows certain listed professions to administer and/or supply those medications listed within the Schedule as part of their professional practice without the need for a prescription, PSD or PGD.

Under Schedule 17, midwives and appropriately supervised student midwives can administer the hepatitis B vaccination.

8.11 Medicines That May Be Administered in Emergency

The legislation (Schedule 19 HMR 2012) allows certain medicines to be administered in an emergency without the directions of a prescriber. In relation to the administration of vaccines, vaccinators need to be specifically aware of this in relation to adrenaline which needs to be given in an emergency in the event of an anaphylactic event following vaccine administration (see Chap. 10). While anaphylaxis after a vaccination is rare, adrenaline must always be available (see Green Book Chap. 8). If it is needed, there is no requirement for any practitioner to have any specific authorisation to administer it. All vaccinators must therefore ensure they are appropriately trained in how and when to use adrenaline and how to manage anaphylaxis against national guidance (Resus Council 2021).

Chapter 9 further discusses best practice in vaccine administration.

8.12 Conclusion

The legal administration of vaccines causes some concern in practice settings. This is often because people do not fully understand the legal requirements and their rationale. This chapter has described the process nurses need to follow in the context of vaccine administration. The ultimate goal of safe and effective medicine supply and administration is to optimise the benefits offered by treatment and achieve the best outcome for each patient; it is an integral part of most nursing and midwifery practice.

Effective medicines management places the patient as the primary focus, thus delivering timely, targeted care and better informed individuals. It is recognised that while the majority of medicines should be prescribed on an individual, patient-specific basis, PGDs offer an advantage to the patient by making vaccines readily accessible without compromising safety and by ensuring there is a robust legal process.

See Box 8.6 for further guidance.

Box 8.6 Further Guidance and Resources

RCN "Medicine supply and administration" resource: https://www.rcn.org.uk/clinical-topics/medicines-management/medicine-supply-and-administration

RCN "Immunisation services delivery": https://www.rcn.org.uk/clinical-topics/Public-health/Immunisation/Immunisation-services-delivery

GP mythbuster 19: Patient Group Directions (PGDs)/Patient Specific Directions (PSDs) https://www.cqc.org.uk/guidance-providers/gps/nigels-surgery-19-patient-group-directions-pgds-patient-specific-directions

(continued)

Box 8.6 (continued)

NICE Medicines Practice Guideline 2 (MPG2) Patient group directions https://www.nice.org.uk/guidance/MPG2
UKHSA national PGD templates: https://www.gov.uk/government/collections/immunisation-patient-group-direction-pgd
Resources from Specialist Pharmacy Services—the first stop for professional medicines advice: https://www.sps.nhs.uk/

- SPS (2024) An introduction to PGDs https://www.sps.nhs.uk/articles/introduction-to-pgds/
- SPS (2024) When to use a PGD https://www.sps.nhs.uk/articles/when-pgds-can-be-used/
- SPS (2024) Patient Specific Directions (PSD): https://www.sps.nhs.uk/articles/patient-specific-directions-psd/
- SPS (2023) Understanding roles and responsibilities of PGD signatories: https://www.sps.nhs.uk/articles/understanding-roles-and-responsibilities-of-pgd-signatories/
- SPS (2024) *Seasonal influenza vaccination and occupational health services* https://www.sps.nhs.uk/articles/seasonal-influenza-vaccination-and-occupational-health-services/
- SPS (2024) PGDs and Occupational Health Services: https://www.sps.nhs.uk/articles/occupational-health-services-ohs-and-medicines-mechanisms/

References

BMA (2019) *The Occupational Physician* British Medical Association, 2019 [Available on line bma_the_occupational_physician_oct_2019.pdf accessed September 2022]
Human Medicines Regulations (2012) http://www.legislation.gov.uk/uksi/2012/1916/contents/made [Accessed September 2022]
Kenny C (2013) Appropriate ways of using PGDs Independent Nurse July 2013 http://www.independentnurse.co.uk/news/appropriate-ways-of-using-pgds/63164 [Accessed September 2022]
Medicines Act Legislation (1968) http://www.legislation.gov.uk/ukpga/1968/67/contents [Accessed September 2022]
MHRA (2017) Patient group directions: who can use them, guidance. https://www.gov.uk/government/publications/patient-group-directions-pgds/patient-group-directions-who-can-use-them [Accessed September 2022]
NICE (2017) Medicines practice guideline [MPG2] Patient Group Directions Overview | Patient group directions | Guidance | NICE [Accessed September 2022]
NMC (2022) The Code: Professional standards of practice and behaviour for nurses, midwives and nursing associates https://www.nmc.org.uk/standards/code/ [Accessed September 2022]
Resus Council (2021): Emergency treatment of anaphylactic reactions: Guidelines for healthcare providers Emergency treatment of anaphylactic reactions: Guidelines for healthcare providers | Resuscitation Council UK [Accessed September 2022]
UKHSA (on line) (n.d.) Immunisation against infectious disease—The Green Book https://www.gov.uk/government/collections/immunisation-against-infectious-disease-the-green-book
UKHSA (2025) Guidance: Quality criteria for an effective immunisation programme https://www.gov.uk/government/publications/quality-criteria-for-an-effective-immunisation-programme (07/07/2025)

Vaccine Administration

9

Michelle Falconer, Pauline MacDonald, Laura Craig, Lesley McFarlane, Debbie Brown, and Jane Dolega-Ossowski

9.1 Introduction

Vaccines may be administered in a number of circumstances:

- To eligible people in the population, as part of routine national vaccination programmes
- To people identified in specific risk groups, either because of underlying medical conditions or due to lifestyle or occupation
- To protect individuals after exposure to an infection (following health protection advice)
- Following a travel health consultation

Vaccines may be live or inactivated and monovalent or multivalent (see Chap. 3). The UK vaccination schedule is comprehensive, and recommendations regarding the vaccines used are subject to frequent changes. Consequently, it is recommended that all immunisers have appropriate training, achieve the recommended competencies and are confident when administering vaccines (UKHSA (2025); NES, 2022).

M. Falconer (✉)
Public Health Scotland (PHS), Edinburgh, UK
e-mail: michellefalconer@aol.com

P. MacDonald
Infection Matters Limited, London, UK
e-mail: macdonald@infectionmatters.com

L. Craig · L. McFarlane
Design, Implementation and Clinical Guidance Division, UK Health Security Agency, London, UK
e-mail: Laura.Craig@ukhsa.gov.uk; lesley.mcfarlane@ukhsa.gov.uk

D. Brown · J. Dolega-Ossowski
London, UK

© Springer Nature Switzerland AG 2025
H. Donovan, H. Bedford (eds.), *Safe Vaccine Administration*,
https://doi.org/10.1007/978-3-031-92498-9_9

National guidance should be used to inform local policy, and systems should be in place to ensure that staff involved in all immunisation programmes have the relevant education and support (see Chap. 4 and Appendix on Scope of Practice). Vaccinators also need to have appropriate authorisation for safe medicines supply and administration (see Chap. 8).

The detail on the UK routine vaccination schedule can be found in the Green Book Chap. 11 (UKHSA online).

9.2 Before the Vaccine Is Delivered

9.2.1 Reducing Procedural Anxiety

For some infants, children, adolescents and adults, the vaccination process can be very stressful, but there are strategies and techniques that a vaccinator can use to reduce stress, minimise pain and provide reassurance (Taddio et al. 2010a, b; WHO, 2015). Being calm, confident, comforting and well-prepared helps to allay people's anxieties, along with using distraction techniques which will be discussed further later in this chapter under positioning and reducing pain.

9.2.2 Informed Consent

Informed consent is required before the administration of any vaccine (see Chap. 7). The individual or the person acting in their best interest and parents or guardians must be given sufficient time to ask questions and the opportunity to discuss the benefits and risks associated with the vaccine being offered, the diseases it protects against and the consequences of not being vaccinated. Developing a trusting relationship with patients, parents or guardians can provide reassurance around the vaccination process and help to increase confidence if they need to return for any follow-up or future vaccinations (see Chap. 6).

Informed consent can be given verbally by the individual—it does not need to be in writing. It must, however, be documented that it was obtained in the clinical record.

9.2.3 Safe Administration

This section incorporates the following:

- Appointment time
- Access to information
- Clinic environment
- Being prepared
- Understanding the schedule and specific patient needs
- Other wider consultation considerations

All the above contribute to safe and effective administration of a vaccine.

Before a vaccine is introduced for use in the UK population, it needs to be licensed, recommendations for use need to be agreed and confirmation of cost-effectiveness needs to be formulated. It can take many years for a vaccine to progress from conception to licensure and production (see Chap. 3). All the years of research work, time and money and the potential protection from the vaccine can be negated if the administration of the vaccine to the eligible individual is not performed correctly.

9.2.4 Appointment Time

Best practice recommendations are for 20 min to be allocated for a childhood vaccination appointment (RCN, 2021), but this may differ depending on the setting where vaccination is taking place, whether staff are available to assist an immuniser with the process, the vaccine recipient's age and the number of vaccines to be given (see Box 9.1).

> **Box 9.1 Key Considerations for Ensuring There Is Enough Time for Vaccine Appointments**
>
> The appointment needs to be long enough to allow an immuniser to
>
> - Provide sufficient information about the vaccines being given and the diseases they protect against
> - Respond to any questions the patient or parent may have
> - Obtain informed consent for each of the vaccines
> - Prepare the vaccines
> - Administer the vaccines
> - Document the vaccines given
> - Provide immediate postvaccination observation and advice
> - Advise on timing of any future doses required to complete a course
>
> Certain scenarios may mean that more time will be needed, and these include the following:
>
> - an infant's first vaccine appointment, so a full assessment, information and support can be given.
> - complex appointments with multiple vaccines and/or additional tests
> - when there is a complicated, uncertain, or unknown vaccination history
> - when the patient or their carer is particularly anxious, hesitant, or concerned
> - when there needs to be careful assessment of a patient's health condition and potential for contraindications (especially for live vaccines)
> - when vaccinating housebound patients

Less time per patient may be required where only one vaccine is being given such as adult influenza and COVID-19 vaccine clinics in GP or pharmacy settings or in vaccination centres. Clinics held in schools may be delivered over several hours with many children being immunised by a school vaccination team during that period.

9.2.5 Clinic Environment

The clinical environment should be safe for both staff and those attending for vaccination. Preparation of the clinic environment is essential to ensure safe administration of vaccines.

- There should be a designated room or area for vaccination clinics/sessions with all the vaccines required for the session stored within the correct temperature range in a designated vaccine fridge (see Chap. 5).
- There should be a clean, clutter-free area for vaccine preparation; a handwashing sink; easy access to disposable equipment required for vaccination, such as needles, syringes and cotton wool; as well as appropriate waste disposal facilities (see Chaps. 10 and 11).
- Access to anaphylaxis equipment including adrenaline and suitable needles and syringes within easy reach. The Resuscitation Council UK (Resus council 2021) has a useful poster and detailed advice on anaphylaxis guidance for vaccination settings (see also Chap. 10).
- Sharps bins, needles, syringes and vaccines should be stored safely out of the reach of children and should be sealed and disposed of in accordance with local policy (see Chap. 11).

9.2.6 Being Prepared

Before commencing the clinic session, confirmation should be made of the vaccines that are required. The clinic list of attendees may assist with this; however, checks should be made that all those attending for vaccination are up to date with any other vaccines for which they are eligible. Additional vaccines may also be recommended for those with underlying health conditions which put them at increased risk from certain diseases (Green Book Chap. 7). Where individuals are not up to date with the vaccines they are eligible for, they should be offered those they are missing in accordance with the UKHSA algorithm "Vaccination of individuals with uncertain or incomplete immunisation status". This document is updated regularly in line with programme changes, and vaccinators are recommended to access the document on line to ensure that they are using the current version.

9.3 Understanding the Schedule and Specific Patient Needs

The current UK immunisation schedule is available in the on line version of the Green Book and in the most up to date version of the UKHSA Complete routine immunisation schedule poster.

9.3.1 Before Administering a Vaccine

- **Check the patient details:**
  Make sure that the right patient is attending for vaccination by checking their personal details and vaccination history. This is particularly important and can be challenging when twins or multiple children are present in the clinic room.
- **Check the records and vaccine history:**
  Any vaccines given previously should be documented in the parent held record (Red Book) and the medical records. As stated, if vaccine status is incomplete, or is unknown, national/local recommendations should be followed, and the guidance in the Green Book along with the most up to date version of the UKHSA "Vaccination of individuals with uncertain or incomplete immunisation status" is used to offer any vaccines they are eligible for.
- **Check for any allergies, contraindications or precautions for the vaccine being given:**
  The person to be vaccinated/parent or guardian should also be asked to describe any previous reactions to vaccines and check that they are well and fit for vaccination.
  Live vaccines are generally contraindicated for patients with immunosuppression—a clinical assessment must be completed which should include a check of any underlying medical condition or treatment that may lead to immunosuppression. If there is any doubt about whether a patient is immunosuppressed, advice should be sought from the clinician providing care/treatment before administering a live vaccine.
- **Administering vaccines together—coadministration:**
  Most vaccines can be given together on the same day at the same appointment. There are some exceptions for certain live vaccines where a specific interval is required to ensure an adequate immune response to each vaccine. There may also be advice against coadministration of other vaccines as a precaution, particularly where vaccines are new to the schedule. This may be to minimise potential adverse reactions or where coadministration may reduce the response to one or both vaccines.
  This will be detailed in the individual vaccine programme, "Information for healthcare practitioners document, the Green Book specific disease chapter and Chap. 11 'UK Immunisation schedule'" (see UKHSA Immunisation collection on line).

9.4 Vaccine Consultation Considerations

- Potential distractions may occur when an extended family and/or noisy active siblings attend for vaccination.
- The assistance of a colleague may be useful in such circumstances to ensure that babies and children are settled comfortably and securely before the procedure.
- Errors can occur in any clinical setting, so it is important to remain vigilant when families, twins or siblings attend for vaccination. When vaccinating several members of the same family, each person should be seen individually if possible. If this is not possible, the help of a colleague should be requested to supervise and check processes.

9.5 Medicines Administration: Best Practice Guidance

Chapter 8 discussed the legislation on medicines administration.

The person administering a medicine needs to follow best practice and know what the medicine is for, how it works, how it should be used and any possible side effects. The standards for best practice on medicines administration are set out on the joint RCN RPS guidance (RCN RPS 2019).

When administering a vaccine, the quick guide in the RCN "Managing childhood immunisation clinics" (RCN 2021) has a useful check list using the 8 Rights (Rs) (Box 9.2).

Box 9.2 The 8 Rs for Vaccine Administration—before Giving A Vaccine, Always Check the Following

1. Right patient
2. Right vaccine and diluent (where applicable)
3. Right to give (i.e. no contraindications)
4. Right time (including correct age and interval, as well as before the product expiration date)
5. Right dose
6. Right route (including correct needle gauge, length and technique)
7. Right site
8. Right documentation (to ascertain what the patient has already had/needs).

9.5.1 Preparing Vaccines

When confident about the vaccines to be given, it has been confirmed there are no contraindications and the parent or appropriate individual has given informed consent, the vaccines can be removed from the fridge and prepared.

Vaccines should only be removed from the fridge and prepared for use when the patient is ready to be vaccinated. This should not be done any earlier as it could lead to errors, unnecessary waste if the vaccines are not required and disruption of the cold chain which could compromise the quality of the vaccine (see Chap. 5).

This section considers the following:

- Needle choice
- Pre-filled syringes, drawing up, reconstituting vaccines and multidose vials
- Skin preparation
- The order in which vaccines are given and general considerations on preparing to give them

9.5.2 Needle Choice

Recommendations on needle size for all routes of injected vaccines are based on studies to ascertain which size of needle provides maximum vaccine effectiveness and reduces local reactions (vaccine reactogenicity). For the majority of intramuscular (IM) vaccines, a 25 mm/23 gauge (blue) needle or 25 mm/25 gauge (orange) needle should be used. It is important that a vaccine designed to be given intramuscularly is delivered into the muscle. Full details of recommendations, rationale and other options for needle size for all injected routes are available in the Green Book Chap. 4, and it is strongly recommended that vaccinators familiarise themselves with these before starting to administer vaccines.

It is important to note that most vaccines used in the UK national programme are supplied with needles either in the box or attached to the syringe. These needles should be used, choosing the most appropriately sized one for administration of the vaccine (Vaccine Update July 2015). When needles are supplied with vaccines, there is no requirement to use needle safe devices for vaccination (Vaccine Update Jan 2016).

Using any needles not supplied with the device or not recommended in the SmPC risks "modification" of the device. Not using the device as supplied is classed as "off-label use" and may count as manufacture of a "new device" under the Medical Devices Regulations (MHRA, 2021).

9.5.3 Pre-filled Syringes

Many pre-filled vaccine syringes are supplied with an integral needle which cannot be removed. Some pre-filled syringes will be supplied with a cap, and the appropriate size of needle or needles will be supplied in the product box; these should be used to administer the vaccine.

An air bubble may be noted in pre-filled vaccine syringes. There is generally no need to expel this air. The action of expelling the air risks losing some of the vaccine. Injecting the air ensures the full dose of vaccine is deposited in the muscle and the needle is cleared (Vaccine Update Nov/Dec 2014). Injecting the air bubble into the muscle may be of some benefit as it can form an airlock in the muscle preventing the vaccine leaking back along the needle track into the subcutaneous tissues which is an event that may result in a stronger localised reaction at the injection site. There may be exceptions and vaccinators should check in the vaccine summary of product characteristics.

9.5.4 Vaccines to Be Drawn up or Reconstituted

Some vaccines may be presented in more than one vial, syringe or ampoule. Although most vaccines in the UK schedule are supplied in single packs, there are some exceptions, for example, COVID-19 vaccine and BCG vaccine are supplied in multidose vials.

It is important to be familiar with recommendations for the preparation of the vaccine and any reconstitution that is required. Details of this procedure will be in the SmPC in the product box. Some vaccines are freeze-dried (lyophilised) and need to be reconstituted before they are administered. Only use the diluent supplied by the manufacturer when reconstituting.

When drawing up vaccines, a 2.5 mL syringe should generally be used unless a very small volume of vaccine is to be given, such as a vaccine dose for intradermal (ID) administration.

The bung on a single dose vaccine vial does not generally need cleaning, and a non-touch technique should suffice. Where multidose vials are used, however, it may be recommended to clean the vial bung before drawing up doses. In general, a green needle (21 G × 38 mm) is recommended to draw up the diluent, to add it to the vaccine and to draw up the vaccine.

When reconstituting a vaccine, the diluent should be added to the vial slowly to prevent frothing and the vaccine gently rotated until the powder has been fully dissolved and the vaccine is fully reconstituted.

Once reconstituted, the vaccine should be inspected to ensure it matches the description given in the SmPC and then administered as soon as possible. If there is any delay, the manufacturer's SmPC should be referred to as different vaccines have different timeframes during which they can be given after reconstitution. Any vaccine which contains visible particles or does not match the description in the SmPC should be discarded in the appropriate waste stream (see Chap. 11).

Once drawn up, the needle should be changed to one of suitable gauge and length or, as provided with the vaccine, before administering the vaccine to the patient.

When a vaccine has been reconstituted, any air bubbles should be expelled from the syringe as it would be difficult to calculate how much air should remain (as seen in pre-filled syringes). Air should be expelled slowly and carefully to ensure that no vaccine is expelled from the tip of the needle as this would result in an incomplete dose being administered. See Figs. 9.1 and 9.2 vaccine preparation.

9 Vaccine Administration

Fig. 9.1 Vaccine preparation

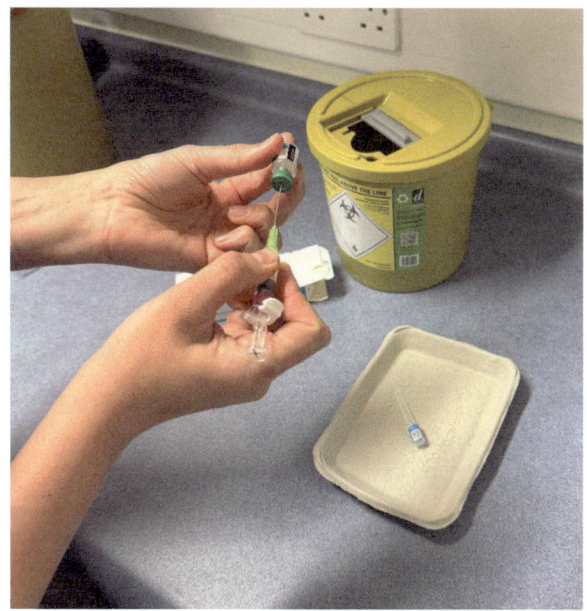

Fig. 9.2 Vaccine preparation

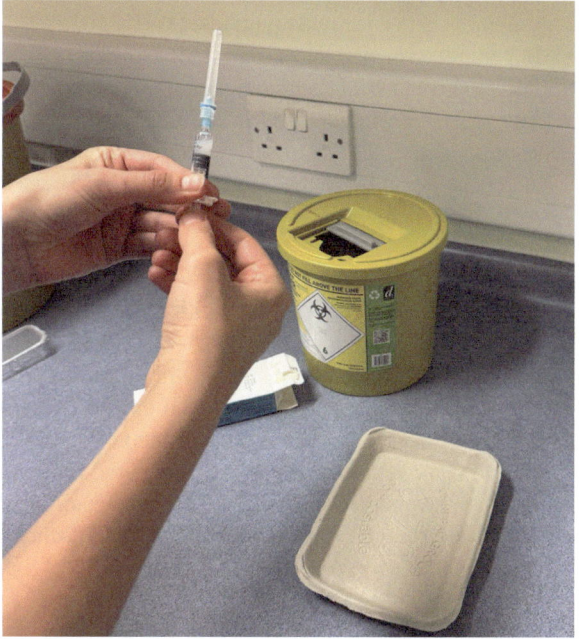

9.5.5 Skin Preparation

Clean skin does not require cleansing prior to vaccination. There is evidence that disinfecting the skin makes no difference to the incidence of bacterial complications from injections (Green Book Chap. 4). If the skin is visibly dirty, it only needs to be washed with soap and water. The use of alcohol and other disinfecting agents could inactivate live vaccines, and they may also cause local irritation if tracked into the muscle when the vaccine is injected.

9.6 Order in Which Vaccines Are Given

Where multiple vaccines are due to be given at the same appointment, there are no absolute requirements, but it often helps to establish a system to minimise the risk of errors. There are some things to consider to help reduce discomfort and aid the process:

- Some vaccines are known to cause more local pain than others. For example, MMR HPV and PCV vaccines have been reported to sting when administered (Ipp et al., 2009).
- It can help to administer vaccines in order of increasing painfulness, giving the vaccines that cause most pain last (WHO 2015).
- In general, oral vaccines are best given before injected vaccines as it is more difficult to give an oral vaccine if the infant is crying following the injected vaccines.
- The rotavirus vaccine used in the UK programme contains sucrose. As there is good evidence that sucrose containing solutions may provide some temporary analgesic effect in infants (Taddio et al., 2015) where it is scheduled to be given, rotavirus vaccine should preferably be administered before the injected vaccines.

9.7 Route and Site of Vaccination

Most of the vaccines administered within the UK national programme are given intramuscularly (IM)—a few are given orally. There are some vaccines and situations where vaccines are given subcutaneously (SC) or intradermally (ID) and the intranasal route is used for the live attenuated influenza vaccine (LAIV). Vaccines must not be given intravenously. Full details regarding their preparation and route of administration can be found in the individual vaccines' SmPC and the disease specific chapters of the Green Book.

9.7.1 Intramuscular (IM) Injections for Individuals with a Bleeding Disorder

Vaccines and similar small volumes of medication can safely be administered via IM injection to people with bleeding disorders. As part of this assessment, consider the following:

- If the individual is on medication to reduce bleeding, for example, treatment for haemophilia. Could the IM vaccine injection be scheduled after the medication or treatment has been given?
- Providing the individual is on stable anticoagulation therapy, including those on warfarin who are up to date with their scheduled international normalized ratio (INR) testing, and the latest INR was below the upper threshold of their therapeutic range, they can receive IM injections.

The guidance recommends a fine needle (equal to 23 gauge or finer calibre such as 25 gauge) should be used followed by firm pressure applied to the site (without rubbing) for at least 2 min and advising the individual that it may bruise.

If in any doubt, consult with the clinician responsible for prescribing or monitoring the individual's anticoagulant therapy. See the Green Book, specific vaccine chapters.

See Table 9.1 for a summary and overview of vaccination routes.

Table 9.1 Vaccination routes

Intramuscular (IM) technique	IM injections should be given with needle at a 90° angle to the skin. The skin should be held flat and not bunched
Subcutaneous (SC) route	For the subcutaneous route, a 25 mm/23-gauge (orange) needle is preferable and should be inserted into the subcutaneous tissue below the dermal layer at an angle of 45° to the skin. To avoid injecting the vaccine into the muscle, it is recommended that the skin is bunched up or pinched to raise the tissues from the muscle layer so that the needle can be inserted into the correct place
Intradermal (ID) technique	The intradermal technique is sometimes used in vaccination. As this route requires a high degree of skill and care, immunisers should ensure they receive specific training and obtain competence in this technique before performing it
Oral route	Giving a vaccine orally may seem like an easy and convenient route; however, oral vaccines need particular and careful preparation. Although only a few vaccines are currently given by this route, it is likely that more will come into the schedule
Nasal route	The live attenuated influenza vaccine (LAIV) is the only UK vaccine currently given by this route. Guidance on how to administer the vaccine is available in the product's SmPC, in the Green Book Chap. 19 and via video produced by NHS Education for Scotland

9.8 Injection Site

The injection site must be chosen based on the optimum route for vaccine efficacy and to avoid risk of damage to nerves, blood vessels or other structures.

The Green Book Chap. 4 "Immunisation Procedures" details this. See Fig. 9.3.

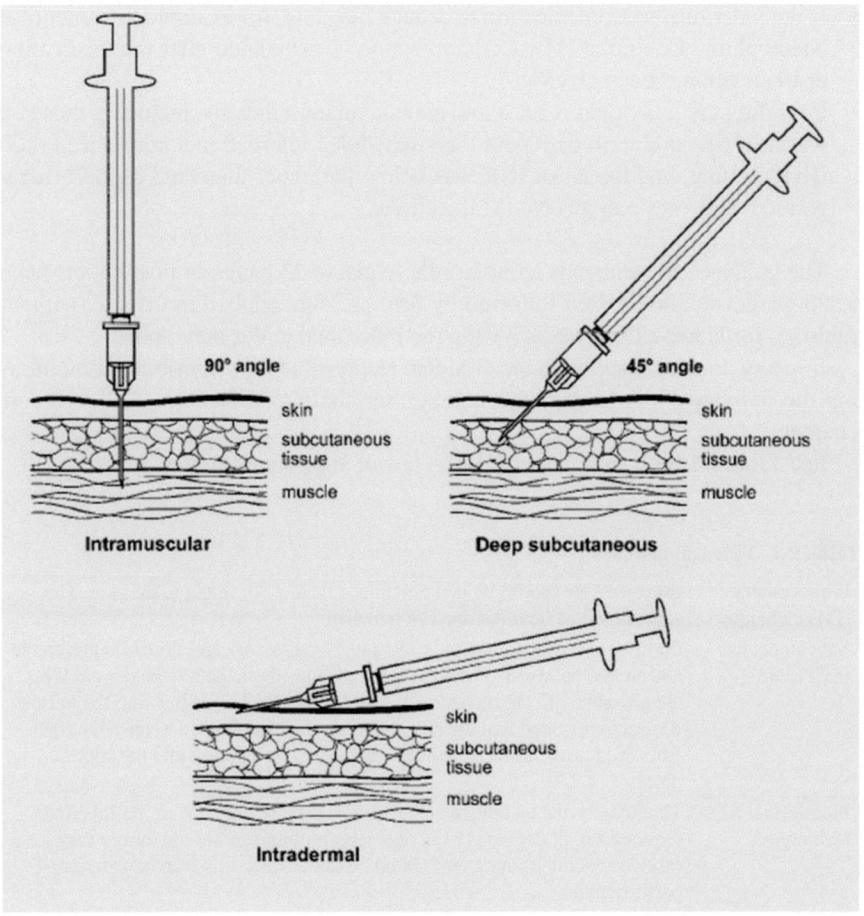

Fig. 9.3 Injection for procedures (Green Book Chap. 4 "Immunisation Procedures")

9.9 Infants Under the Age of 1 Year

All intramuscular vaccinations must be given in the anterolateral aspect of the thigh (vastus lateralis muscle), which provides a large muscle mass. Incorrectly injecting into the upper surface (anterior aspect) of the thigh risks injecting into fat, nerves and blood vessels, so care should be taken to avoid this.

The deltoid muscle is not generally used in infants as it is not sufficiently developed at this age. Infants should be undressed down to their nappy so that the whole thigh, hip and knee can be visualised. The immuniser can then be sure not to give the vaccine too high or too low on the thigh. It may be particularly important to visualise all the anatomy if two vaccines need to be given in the thigh as a 2.5 cm gap should be left between them and the site of administration for each vaccine clearly documented. This will enable identification of each vaccine in the event of a local reaction. See Fig. 9.4 (also see the sections below on giving multiple vaccines and positioning and reducing pain).

Exceptions: If the anterolateral aspect of the thigh is not accessible in an infant, for example, if they attend for vaccination while in a spica cast, consideration will need to be given as to whether it would be possible to administer the vaccine during a cast change, whether a window could be cut in the cast to enable vaccine

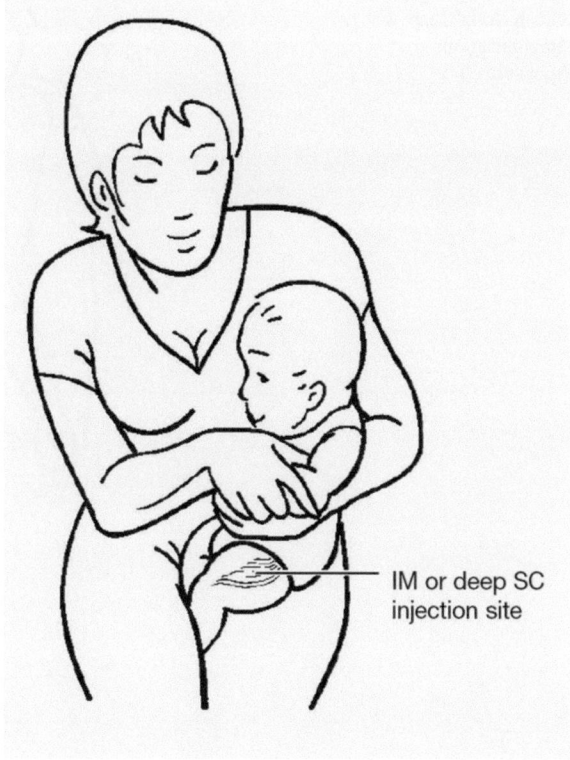

Fig. 9.4 Preferred site for intramuscular and deep subcutaneous injections in infants under 1 year of age (Green Book Chap. 4 "Immunisation Procedures")

administration or whether the deltoid muscle may be the only accessible site at this time. As the location of the radial nerve is more superficial in infants, additional consideration will need to be given to the needle size and injection technique used (Australian Government Department of Health 2021).

9.10 For Children over the Age of 12 Months and Adults

The deltoid muscle in the upper arm can be used for IM injections as well as the thigh. At the 12-month visit, when more vaccines may be needed to be given, all limbs may be used. For older children and adults, the deltoid muscle is the preferred injection site as it is easier to access and provides sufficient muscle mass (see Figs. 9.5, 9.6, and 9.7).

Figures 9.3, 9.4, and 9.5 taken from the Green Book Chap. 4 "Immunisation Procedures" UK Health Security Agency. Content available under the Open Government Licence v3.0

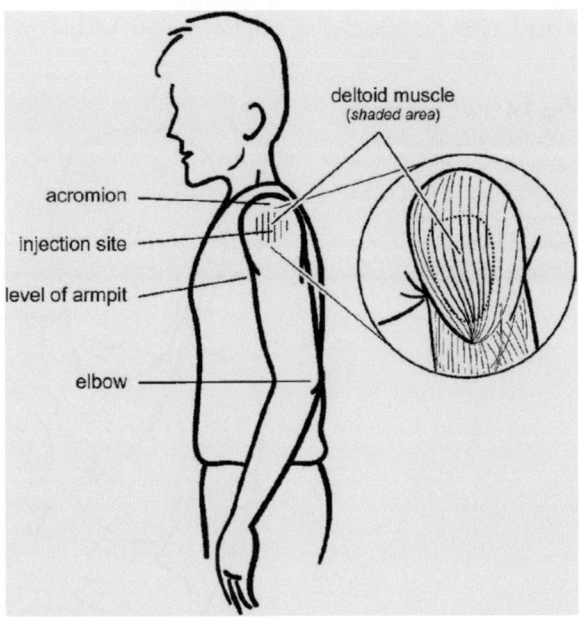

Fig. 9.5 Preferred site for intramuscular and deep subcutaneous injections in older children and adults (Green Book Chap. 4 "Immunisation Procedures")

Fig. 9.6 IM injection being given in deltoid in a child

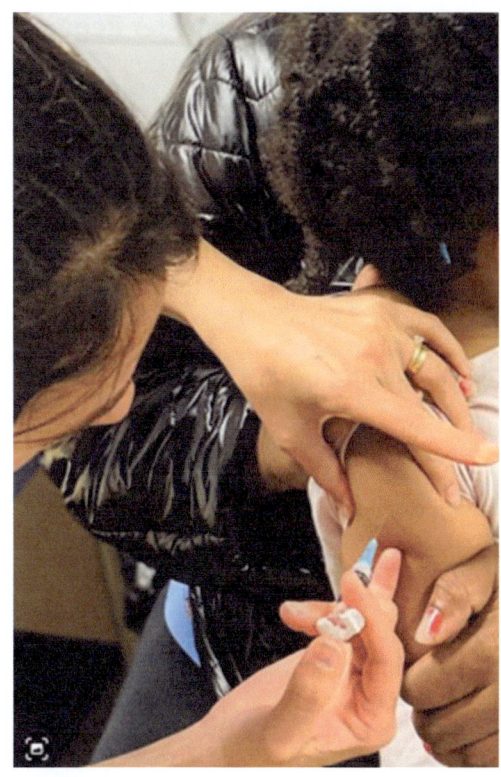

Fig. 9.7 IM injection being given in deltoid in an adult

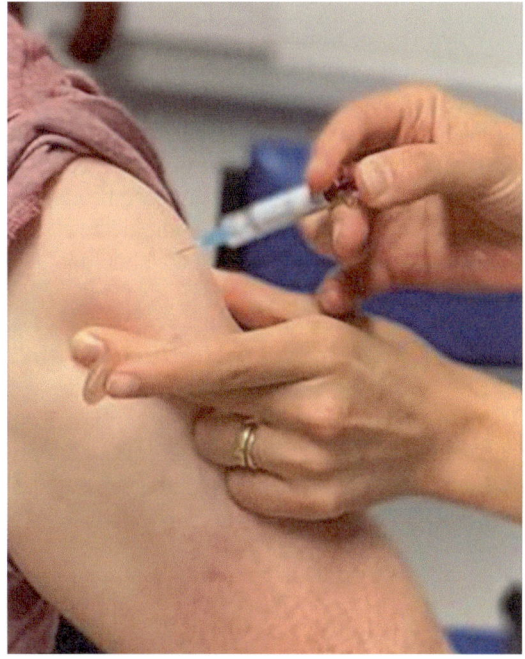

9.11 Cautions to Consider Regarding Vaccine Site

- Do not inject vaccines into the buttocks as there is a risk of sciatic nerve damage and injecting into fatty tissue will reduce vaccine immunogenicity.
- It may be better to avoid injecting vaccines into limbs where there is risk of lymphoedema or where recent surgery has taken place wherever possible. See NHS lymphoedema prevention https://www.nhs.uk/conditions/lymphoedema/prevention/.
- Vaccines must not be administered into the arm where BCG vaccination has been given for 3 months afterward due to the risk of regional lymphadenitis (Green Book Chap. 32).
- It is essential that the correct site and injection technique is used to administer vaccines. Injecting too high into the upper arm might result in a shoulder injury or a frozen shoulder. This leads to pain, weakness and a limited range of motion that can last for months. Injecting too low or too far to the side of the arm risks injecting into the axillary nerve or the radial nerve. To avoid shoulder injury, always assess the limb before administering the vaccine to identify the correct site for injection.
- When new vaccines are introduced into the routine schedule, there is often a national recommendation to give them into a specified limb. Following these recommendations as closely as possible facilitates more accurate recording and reporting of any local adverse reactions caused by the newly introduced vaccine.

9.12 Giving Multiple Vaccines

- When two or more injections need to be administered, they should be given in separate sites and preferably into different limbs.
- If two or more vaccines need to be given in the same limb, then they should be given 2.5 cm apart (Green Book Chap. 4; American Academy of Paediatrics 2003).
- The specific sites should be documented so that if there are any extensive local reactions, the causative vaccine can be easily identified.
- The exact site of each vaccine should be clearly documented, for example, noting "nearest the hip" or "nearest the shoulder".

9.13 Positioning and Reducing Pain

Using distraction techniques as appropriate for the person's age during the procedure can help reduce pain and minimise the individual's anxiety, for example, talking about interests, using breathing techniques or using toys, music or bubble blowing.

9.13.1 Infants and Children

The infant should be held securely, so that the limb to be injected does not move during the vaccination process to prevent vaccination errors or needle stick injuries (WHO 2015) (Fig. 9.8). Be mindful, however, that being held too tightly may convey excess anxiety and fear to the child.

Parents should be advised to hold their infant in a position that feels comfortable and natural for them and that is comfortable for the child while allowing for effective holding of the limbs to facilitate safe vaccination.

If a parent is very anxious, it may be necessary for another member of staff to assist by holding the child during the procedure.

Explaining the procedure to young children (with agreement from their parents/carers) in simple language that they can understand can also help to reduce surprise and future distrust.

9.14 Practical Guidelines. Based on "Reducing Pain During Vaccine Injections: Clinical Practice Guideline" (Taddio et al. 2015)

- Caregivers should hold the infant or child securely on their lap with the limbs to be injected held firmly and the other limbs held safely out the way.
- For older children, make an assessment about how confidently they will respond to the process, and use a caregiver to hold them securely when possible.
- Breast-feeding infants can be fed for comfort during or following vaccinations (see Fig. 9.9).

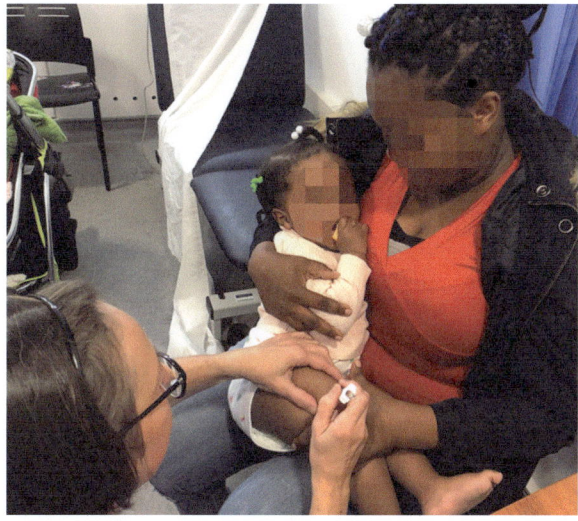

Fig. 9.8 Parent holding infant securely for the vaccine administration

Fig. 9.9 Image showing mother breast-feeding during the vaccination

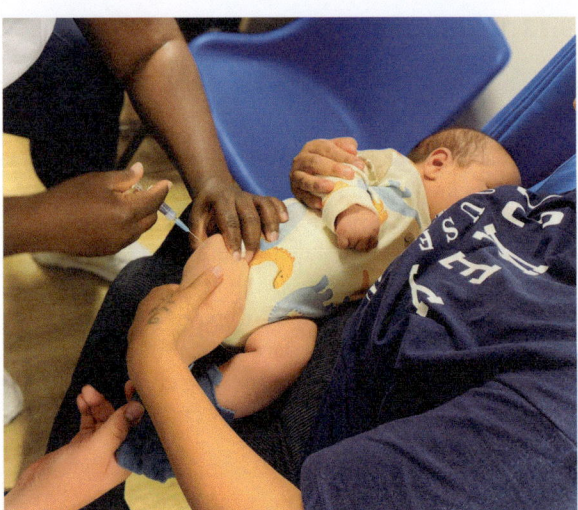

- For younger children, use distraction such as music, toys, etc.
- Offer rewards such as stickers to children after vaccination.
- Don't spend too long cajoling children into having their vaccination. This is not effective and can lead to heightened distress and delay the consultation time. Get the caregivers to collaborate with you and help develop the child's trust in the process.
- Ultimately, vaccinating the child is a valuable and important process, and short-term pain and distress may be unavoidable. Most children will cry but will usually settle quickly once the procedure is completed.

Figure 9.10 is based on the information.

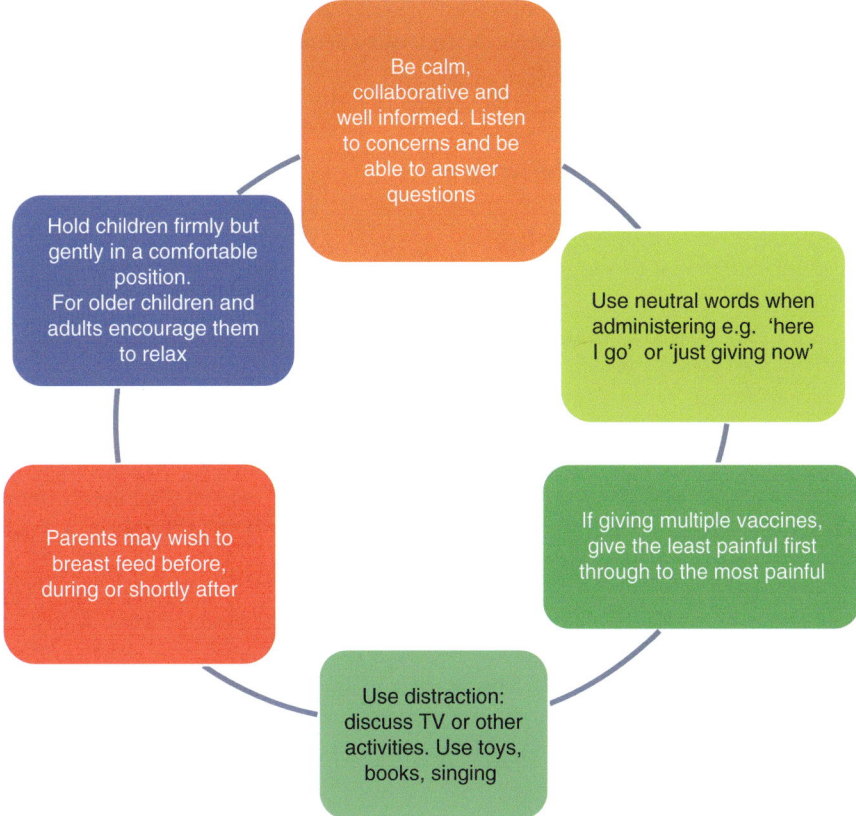

Fig. 9.10 Key areas to help minimise discomfort during vaccination

9.15 Teenagers and Adults

Fainting can be common in adolescents after vaccination and can lead to injury (CDC, 2015). Each patient's potential for fainting should be assessed by asking about their previous experiences of having vaccinations and assessing their feelings and attitudes toward the process, being mindful of signs of anxiety such as hyperventilation, weakness, pallor and sweating. It is good practice to ensure patients are sitting down, and, in some cases, it may be best to advise them to lie on a couch while they relax their arm on their lap, tabletop or couch.

Distraction techniques such as conversation about topics of interest, providing an explanation of the process, encouraging relaxation, suggesting wiggling of toes and suggesting breathing techniques, i.e. cough as the needle is inserted (WHO, 2015), can all help to reduce anxiety.

Dishonesty such as "this won't hurt" (WHO 2015) and using terms such as "sharp scratch coming" may heighten anxiety, so using calm, neutral words such as "here we go" is preferable.

Teenagers and adults can also be advised to bring a friend or family member to the appointment for additional support.

See Box 9.3 for some useful resources.

Box 9.3 Resources to Support Reducing Anxiety and Minimising Pain During Vaccination

A number of resources have been developed to support COVID-19 vaccination. The general principles advocated in these resources apply to all age groups during vaccination.

- The British Psychological Society—support for children and young people having a blood test or vaccination (Mackay, 2022).
- Elearning for healthcare (Elfh) hosts a module "Paediatric procedural anxiety module for COVID-19 vaccinations" from Great Ormond St Elfh portal.
- NHS England—Top tips for supporting children and young people during vaccination.
- TURAS NHS Education for Scotland (NES) Supporting vaccination reducing procedural anxiety and pain. Includes eLearning, slides and a poster for both adults and children.
- NHS Wales—Distraction techniques to minimise a child's anxiety during vaccination.
- SAPHNA Guidance: children, young people and needle phobia | SAPHNA—School And Public Health Nurses Association https://saphna.co/news/saphna-guidance-children-young-people-and-needle-phobia/.
- Canadian government advice Vaccination pain management for children: Guidance for health care providers.

Box 9.4 provides further general vaccine administration tips.

Box 9.4 General Vaccine Administration Tips

The general principle is to make the procedure safe but as quick and as uncomplicated as possible to minimise the pain and general anxiety often associated with having a vaccine.

The WHO position paper "Reducing pain at the time of vaccination: WHO position paper –2015" considered the pros and cons of many aspects of vaccine administration.

(continued)

Box 9.4 (continued)

1. The use of topical anaesthetic before vaccination may be effective and tempting, but they complicate the procedure unnecessarily, increasing the appointment time and the cost of the vaccination procedure, and as such are not routinely recommended.
2. It is not necessary to rub the injection site before or after vaccination.
3. Avoid injecting into any areas of broken skin. Although there is a lack of evidence for avoiding injecting into a tattoo (IAC, 2020; Kluger (2021) recommends avoiding vaccinating on a tattoo which is still healing and advising people to avoiding tattooing over a site where a vaccine has recently been administered.
4. The small volumes being injected mean there is no need to aspirate (draw back on the syringe plunger after needle insertion to check for blood). There are no large blood vessels at the recommended injection sites, and there is no evidence that vaccines have accidently been given intravenously. It can also be more uncomfortable and distressing for the vaccine recipient as it extends the time it takes to give the injection and increases the risk of moving the needle sideways (Taddio et al. 2010a, b).
5. Give the injection rapidly and withdraw the needle quickly. Studies have found that this technique is less painful than slow insertion and aspiration followed by slow withdrawal (Ipp et al., 2007).
6. If the injected vaccine leaks and the dose is only partially administered, discount this dose and repeat it at the same appointment (UKHSA 2022).
7. If the recipient moves or pulls away when a needle has passed through the skin, but the vaccine has not been injected, change the needle to re-administer, or, if necessary, discard the vaccine and start afresh.
8. Remove the needle quickly and apply gentle pressure at the injection site with cotton wool or gauze. There is generally no need to use a plaster or to leave the cotton wool in place with tape, unless there is obvious bleeding.

9.16 Postvaccination Advice

This is further considered and discussed in Chap. 10.

It is important to inform the patient or carer about any potential vaccine reactions they might experience and what action to take to prevent or treat them should they occur. This should be backed up with written leaflets specific to the vaccine and or the Patient Information Leaflet (PIL) which comes with the vaccine. For children, the "What to expect after vaccinations" leaflet published by UKHSA and a similar leaflet What to expect after immunisation—babies and children up to 5 from NHS inform Scotland can be used.

It can be helpful to explain that as vaccines produce an immune response, this can result in short lasting effects such as soreness and pain at the injection site, feeling achy and lethargic, and, in some cases, a fever.

Ensure the patient/carer knows when the next vaccinations are due; provide a leaflet or written information if possible. It is good practice to provide this even if they say they have the information at home. Giving them the information at the time of vaccination increases the opportunity for them to read it and ensure they have it to hand.

Generally, there is no requirement for the recipient to wait for any period of time after their routine vaccinations. However, when new vaccines are introduced, it may be recommended that patients are observed for a specific time after vaccination, for example, for some COVID vaccines, a 15-min observation period was initially advised, but this advice was suspended once more safety data became available. Individuals should be observed initially while they are being given postvaccination information (see Chap. 10), and unless there is a particular history of allergy, no further observation is routinely recommended. Observing postvaccination specifically for anaphylaxis is unfounded and not practical since anaphylaxis can occur at any time up to 72 hours after exposure to an allergen or trigger.

9.17 Record-Keeping and Documentation

There may be a requirement to ensure that the vaccines given are recorded on the local/regional/national child health information system, so it is important to ensure that all records are completed (e.g. child's parent held record or "Red Book", medical records or the vaccine management tool (VMT) for certain vaccines in Scotland).

Some general practice systems will automatically link to the child health information system (CHIS), so once recorded on the GP system, the details will appear on the CHIS. Not all systems or providers have this facility, so vaccinators may need to ensure that this information reaches the CHIS and the patient's GP by other means which include completed clinic sheets/paperwork, email or electronic transfer.

The patient's GP holds their complete health record and therefore should be notified of vaccines given by other providers. It is therefore important that, for patient safety and for accurate measurements of uptake, all the necessary information and correct codes and data are entered unto the systems.

Full details of vaccination procedures can be found in the Green Book Chap. 4.

References

American Academy of Paediatrics (2003). Active Immunisation. In: Pickering LK (ed) Red Book: 2003 Report of the Committee on Infectious Diseases, 26th Edition. Elk. Grove Village, IL: American Academy of Paediatrics, P33

CDC (2015). Fainting (Syncope). Accessed at https://www.cdc.gov/vaccinesafety/concerns/fainting.html

Immunization Action Coalition. 2020. Administering vaccines. https://www.immunize.org/askexperts/administering-vaccines.asp Accessed 03 July 2023

Ipp M, Taddio A, Sam J, Goldbach M, Parkin PC (2007). Vaccine related pain: Randomized controlled trial of two injection techniques. *Arch Dis Child.* 92: 1105-1108 Accessed at https://www.ncbi.nlm.nih.gov/pmc/articles/PMC2066084/

Ipp M, Parkin PC, Lear N, Goldbach M, Taddio A. (2009) Order of vaccine injection and infant pain response. Arch Pediatr Adolesc Med. May;163(5):469-72. https://doi.org/10.1001/archpediatrics.2009.35. PMID: 19414694. Available at: Order of Vaccine Injection and Infant Pain Response | Infectious Diseases | JAMA Pediatrics | JAMA Network Accessed 03 July 2023

Kluger N. (2021) Is it safe to vaccinate within a tattoo? Ann Dermatol Venereol. Dec;148(4):256-258. https://doi.org/10.1016/j.annder.2021.04.008. Epub 2021 Jul 1. PMID: 34218936; PMCID: PMC8248893. Available at Is it safe to vaccinate within a tattoo? - PMC (nih.gov) Accessed 03 July 2023

Mackay F (2022) Supporting children aged 5+ and young people having a blood test or vaccination The British psychological society Supporting children aged 5+ and young people having a blood test or vaccination

NES NHS Education for Scotland, Public Health Scotland (2022). Proficiency dicument for addministration of vaccines by registered health care practitioners NES and PHS TURAS https://learn.nes.nhs.scot/61565

MHRA (2021): Managing Medical Devices. Guidance for Health and social care organisations. https://www.gov.uk/government/publications/managing-medical-devices [Accessed September 2024]

NHS Lymphoedema - Prevention - NHS (n.d.) (www.nhs.uk) https://www.nhs.uk/conditions/lymphoedema/prevention/

NHS England (n.d.) Top tips for supporting children and young people during vaccination https://www.england.nhs.uk/south/wp-content/uploads/sites/6/2021/09/covid-19-top-tips-for-supporting-children-and-young-people-during-vaccination-v1-090821.pdf

NHS Wales Distraction techniques to minimise a child's anxiety during vaccination Distraction techniques to minimise a child's anxiety during vaccination (nhs.wales)

RCN (2021). Managing Childhood Immunisation Clinics. Accessed at Managing Childhood Immunisation Clinics | Royal College of Nursing (rcn.org.uk)

RCN RPS (2019) Professional Guidance on the Administration of Medicines in Healthcare Settings. https://www.rpharms.com/Portals/0/RPS%20document%20library/Open%20access/Professional%20standards/SSHM%20and%20Admin/Admin%20of%20Meds%20prof%20guidance.pdf?ver=2019-01-23-145026-567 [Accessed September 2024]

Resus Council (2021): Anaphylaxis guidance for vaccination settings https://www.resus.org.uk/about-us/news-and-events/anaphylaxis-guidance-vaccination-settings [Accessed June 2023]

Taddio A, Appleton M, Bortolussi R et al (2010a). Reducing the pain of childhood vaccination: an evidence-based clinical practice guideline. *CMAJ.* **182** (18). E843-855. Accessed at https://www.cmaj.ca/content/182/18/E843/tab-figures-data

Taddio A, Flanders D, Weinberg E, et al (2015). Comparison of oral sucrose solution and oral rotavirus vaccine for reducing pain during infant vaccine injections. *Paediatric Child Health* Vol 20 No 5 Accessed at https://academic.oup.com/pch/article/20/5/e97/2649104

UKHSA (2022) Vaccine incident guidance: responding to vaccine errors Accessed July 2023 https://www.gov.uk/government/publications/vaccine-incident-guidance-responding-to-vaccine-errors

UKHSA (2025). National Minimum Standards and Core Curriculum for Vaccination Training https://www.gov.uk/government/publications/national-minimum-standards-and-core-curriculum-for-immunisation-training-for-registered-healthcare-practitioners

WHO (2015). WHO position paper on reducing pain at time of vaccination – Accessed July 2023 https://www.who.int/publications/i/item/who-wer9039

Yin H C, Cheng S W, Yang C Y, Chiu, Y W et al (2017). Comparative Survey of Holding Positions for Reducing Vaccination Pain in Young Infants. *Pain research & management*. 3273171. Accessed at https://www.ncbi.nlm.nih.gov/pmc/articles/PMC5299184/

Taddio A, Appleton A, Bortolussi R et al (2010b). Reducing the pain of childhood vaccination: an evidence-based clinical practice guideline. CMAJ. 182 (18) E843-E855. Accessed at https://www.cmaj.ca/content/182/18/E843.full

Clinic Management

10

Pauline MacDonald and Lesley McFarlane

10.1 The Importance of Quality Vaccination Clinic Management

Much of the research around what works to improve the uptake of vaccines centres on the characteristics and activities of the provider organisation, as opposed to the characteristics and actions of potential vaccine recipients.

Two studies concerned with increasing influenza vaccination rates provide evidence of the independent factors associated with higher vaccine uptake (Dexter et al., 2012; Newby et al., 2016).

Although conducted using different methods, and a few years apart, the results were similar, as presented in Box 10.1.

P. MacDonald (✉)
Infection Matters Limited, London, UK
e-mail: macdonald@infectionmatters.com

L. McFarlane
Design, Immunisation and Clinical Guidance Division, UK Health Security Agency, London, UK

© Springer Nature Switzerland AG 2025
H. Donovan, H. Bedford (eds.), *Safe Vaccine Administration*,
https://doi.org/10.1007/978-3-031-92498-9_10

> **Box 10.1 Key Factors for Quality Vaccine Clinic Management**
> - Clinical leadership,
> - Personal invitations for eligible patients
> - Effective communication
> - Setting targets for performance
> - Good use of IT systems and opportunistic vaccination
>
> These are shown to result in higher vaccine uptake, and each will be addressed in detail in this chapter.

These factors can be applied to all vaccination programmes, whether for influenza vaccine, childhood, adolescent, adult, or even for mass vaccination delivery such as for the COVID-19 vaccines. All these elements are also recommended in the NICE guidance NG218: Vaccine uptake in the general population (NICE, 2022).

The NICE guidance (2022) gives recommendations for commissioners, providers and users of vaccination services and supports the previously published NICE guidance on increasing flu vaccination uptake (NG103 Flu vaccination: increasing uptake dated 22 August 2018 https://www.nice.org.uk/guidance/ng103).

Each vaccinator should be familiar with the NICE guidance on vaccination, as it pertains to their particular service provision. It is sensible to consider the management of individual vaccination clinics in the light of this guidance. The UKHSA Quality criteria for an effective Immunisation programme, states that vaccines need to be given within the regulatory framework for medicines administration (UKHSA 2025a), this chapter describes what these are.

10.2 Knowing the Target Population

In general, knowing the target population for vaccination services is a principal factor for planning vaccination offers and clinics and maximising uptake among that population. Knowing the demographic makeup of the population to be served should be factored into the "who, how, what, when, where and why" of the vaccination offer.

Some population groups have historically low vaccination uptake. The provider of the vaccination service should assess whether their target population includes any of these. Chap. 12 "Maximising Uptake: A Population Approach" discusses this topic in more detail and the need to tailor vaccination clinics and the methods for offering vaccines accordingly.

Vaccinators need to be mindful of the barriers to vaccination (Box 10.2) and deliver vaccination clinics with the aim of overcoming these barriers.

> **Box 10.2 (From NICE May 2022) Some Key Barriers to Routine Vaccine Uptake**
> - Inflexible and inconvenient clinic times and locations
> - Perceived lack of balanced vaccine information (including misinformation)
> - Language and literacy problems
> - Insufficient time in consultations to discuss concerns about vaccinations
> - Lack of staff training in how to discuss vaccinations effectively
> - Uncertainty about vaccine safety and effectiveness
> - Uncertainty about whether vaccines are needed (including how severe the diseases are or how likely it is that someone will be exposed to the disease)
> - Previous negative experiences of vaccination
> - Lack of trust in the government, drug companies and the healthcare system
> - Religious or cultural views that are against vaccination (this may relate to specific vaccinations, for example, HPV [human papillomavirus])
> - Individual barriers such as needle phobia or sensory impairment

This chapter discusses best practice to improve uptake into the context of clinic management at provider level.

10.3 Best Practice for Clinic Management

10.3.1 Leadership

An important influencing factor in high-quality vaccination service delivery is that each provider has a named vaccination lead. The benefit of such a leader is highlighted in research (Dexter et al., 2012; Newby et al., 2016) and is included under the first service organisation recommendation "Leadership" in the NICE guidance NG218 (NICE, 2022). It is recognised that without a named lead, vaccine related services may not be prioritised or satisfactorily completed, especially in the climate of many competing priorities for an organisation.

Having a named lead for vaccination is now a core part of NHS general practice contracts for providing vaccination and immunisation services.

The NICE guidance suggests the responsibilities of the named lead (Box 10.3). It is not their role to personally perform all these elements, but to ensure all team members work together, using their specific skills, expertise and resources to deliver high-quality vaccination services.

> **Box 10.3 Named Vaccination Lead (NICE, 2022)**
> Ensure that each organisation commissioning, providing or organising vaccination services has a named vaccination lead with responsibility (as relevant) for ensuring the following:
>
> - Vaccination records are validated and updated.
> - People who are eligible for vaccination are identified.
> - Invitations and reminders are sent to people eligible for vaccination.
> - Vaccines are administered and recorded.
> - There is coordination between providers and other services involved in organising and reporting vaccinations.
> - GP practices and child health information services (CHIS) understand each other's reporting systems and processes.
> - Best practice is followed for ordering, storing, distributing and disposing of vaccines (see Chap. 5 and the Green Book Chap. 3 for more information).

Each vaccinator should know who the vaccination lead is and be confident that their overall service delivery provides the best opportunity for the target audience to access vaccination. Service delivery and clinic management arrangements should be led by the vaccination lead with continuous review, input and involvement of all those who can influence service delivery. This would include staff both in and outside the organisation and patient or client groups who can help inform population needs and service delivery options. Wide consultation will enable sound clinic management solutions which are suitable for the target population.

If a vaccinator considers that services could be offered more safely, differently or more efficiently, this should be discussed with the vaccination lead. Any safety concerns should always be raised in writing.

Once service provision arrangements at organisational level have been optimised, vaccinators can then turn their attention to the detail of how they and their organisation prepares for, conducts and follows up after vaccination events.

Considering best practice when managing vaccination clinics ensures patient safety is at the heart of the process while also ensuring safety for the vaccinator. Well-organised, calm and efficient vaccination clinics will promote recipient confidence in both the vaccines being offered and the vaccinator. The Royal College of Nursing document "Managing Childhood Immunisation Clinics" (RCN, 2021) provides a clear succinct summary of best practice; all the principles can be applied to all vaccination clinics not just those for children. Vaccinators do well to compare their clinic arrangements with the recommended best practice described in this document.

10.4 Prior to the Clinic

10.4.1 Setting up the Clinics/Appointments

Each vaccination provider organisation may have different target populations, delivery systems and venues at which to vaccinate individuals. When planning vaccination sessions, it is important to consider how easily eligible individuals can access the service. Easy access to vaccination is a key factor in vaccine acceptance and high uptake.

At general practice level, this might be by offering clinics at the practice venue, a community venue in conjunction with other practices in a primary care network, or offering opportunistic vaccination outside a specified clinic time at the practice venue.

For some eligible groups, access to vaccination may be better provided if offered to them in a venue such as their school or workplace, a local convenient community venue, their care or residential home or as domiciliary vaccination at home. All vaccination opportunities need to be planned taking account of the size of the eligible cohort, the window of opportunity or time limitations on specific programmes, the best time of day, length of the appointment time per person, expected levels of demand and nonattendance, vaccine supplies, transport and storage at the venue, management of waste, ability to access medical records and record vaccination activity and staffing levels including expertise and skills.

Consider the environment where the vaccine is to be given—ideally it should be in a private space where people can discuss and ask questions and feel able to remove enough clothing to be able to access the correct injection site. In mass settings, such as schools or office spaces, consider use of screens to give people a private space.

10.4.2 Capturing Vaccination Event Data

Ideally the data pertaining to vaccination delivered outside general practice needs to reach the patient health record, held by their registered GP. By reporting vaccination events to national vaccination measurement systems such as Child Health Information Systems (CHIS), and any other national immunisation data collection systems. The data will be accessible to the patient's registered GP and can then be included in the patient record. The ability to measure vaccination activity is important for assessment of individual protection and planning future vaccination offers to those individuals. It is also crucial for ongoing assessment of the impact of the national vaccination programmes on incidence and outcomes of the vaccine preventable diseases. These data, collected at national level, are used to measure the safety and acceptability of vaccines and informs assessment of required adjustments to the programme in terms of eligible groups, booster requirements or vaccines used.

10.4.3 Vaccines to Be Offered

Before the vaccination clinic, the vaccinator should check the clinic schedule (for prebooked appointments).

- Check which patients have been invited for which vaccines.
- Does the schedule make sense.
- Have they been invited for the vaccines expected for their age and eligibility?
- Are the vaccines available or might they need to be ordered? (Chap. 5 gives more details on vaccine ordering, delivery, storage and stock control).

For both scheduled and opportunistic vaccination delivery, the vaccinator should check the following:

- The patient records and/or any documentation regarding their previous vaccination history and consider if the individual is up to date with all their routine vaccines

If it is thought that individuals may be missing vaccines for which they are eligible, the UKHSA algorithm "Vaccination of individuals with uncertain or incomplete immunisation status" (https://www.gov.uk/government/publications/vaccination-of-individuals-with-uncertain-or-incomplete-immunisation-status) will assist in deciding which vaccines could be offered to which individuals.

In some circumstances, it may be necessary to refer the individual to another provider for missing vaccines, depending on the service provision and contractual arrangements. This may be required if the individual is noted, by a school age immunisation service, to be missing vaccines and is then required to see their GP for missing doses.

The vaccinator should always document the efforts made to establish the recipient's previous vaccination history, which vaccines were offered and for which vaccines an eligible patient gave their consent. This process can often take a lot of time and requires a high degree of vaccination experience and knowledge. Vaccinators should ensure they have protected time for this important part of the assessment and the opportunity to consult with colleagues or access to immunisation advice at local level.

10.4.4 Vaccine Contraindications and Precautions

Familiarity with the vaccines to be offered is important and comes with training, education and experience. As with any medicine, if vaccinators are not totally familiar with a vaccine being offered, they must check the details, product content, indications and contraindications available in the Summary of Product

Characteristics (SmPC) sheet and the relevant chapter of the Green Book—"Immunisation Against Infectious Disease" (https://www.gov.uk/government/collections/immunisation-against-infectious-disease-the-green-book). Only once the vaccinator is knowledgeable, confident and competent to administer a particular vaccine can it be given.

Once the vaccinator is confident that the vaccines being offered are appropriate for the recipient, the medical records and completed consent form, if available in advance of the clinic, should be checked for any contraindications, precautions or allergies to vaccine ingredients. Useful resources to check for vaccine contraindications, precautions and vaccine ingredients are as follows:

- Summary of Product Characteristics sheets are produced for every licensed vaccine. Most vaccine SmPCs are available at the Electronic Medicines Compendium website (https://www.medicines.org.uk/emc).
- The Green Book "Immunisation Against Infectious Disease" chapters on each vaccine preventable disease and vaccine https://www.gov.uk/government/collections/immunisation-against-infectious-disease-the-green-book.
- General information about vaccine ingredients and why they are contained in vaccines can be found at the Oxford Vaccine Group website https://vk.ovg.ox.ac.uk/vaccine-ingredients.

Deciding which vaccines a patient is eligible for and suitable to receive can be challenging. Each vaccine has contraindications and precautions, and each recipient has their individual medical history, questions and concerns. For operational guidance, many of the routine vaccination programmes have accompanying UKHSA documents entitled "Information for Healthcare Professionals/Practitioners". These documents are extensive and will provide answers to almost every question a vaccinator might have regarding day-to-day delivery of the relevant vaccine to eligible individuals. Each national vaccination programme and related supporting documents can be accessed via the Immunisation Collection on GOV.UK website https://www.gov.uk/government/collections/immunisation.

10.4.5 Legal Framework for Administration

Vaccines are prescription only medicines, and vaccinators should ensure there is a legal prescription or framework in place for their administration. The legal framework should be in place before the clinic or vaccination event to support timeliness of vaccination (see Chap. 8 for further detail).

10.5 During the Clinic

10.5.1 Human Resources and Arrangements

Vaccination services are busy, time consuming and relentless, with a constant stream of eligible patients entering the routine vaccination programmes. Consideration of resources available for delivering vaccination clinics is important.

Registered healthcare professionals (HCPs) who are trained and competent to vaccinate do not need to have another immuniser in the building when they are vaccinating, nor does there need be a doctor in the building. However, it is best practice for there to be another person available who can aid and summon help in an emergency.

For domiciliary vaccination, a trained and competent HCP can visit alone to vaccinate. There may be other circumstances, following a risk assessment, which might mean more than one person attends someone at home and all staff should be supported by a loan worker policy or procedure to ensure their safety. The vaccinator must be up to date with training on basic life support and the management of anaphylaxis, as well as having an anaphylaxis kit available when vaccines are administered in any setting.

Healthcare support workers (HCSWs) work at the direction of HCPs and perform delegated tasks and therefore should in turn be supported by registered colleagues. HCSWs who are trained and competent to vaccinate may work alone in their clinic room at their place of employment. It is best practice to ensure that there is appropriate support for the HCSW; they should not be expected to vaccinate in settings without such support. Ideally this should be an HCP, who is also trained and competent to vaccinate, is always accessible and is preferably with them in the building (UKHSA 2025a, b; RCN, 2022).

10.5.2 Length of Vaccination Appointment

Vaccinators should ensure that they have enough time to work safely and are not disturbed by other colleagues or tasks. Unfortunately, vaccination errors occur every day in the UK. Many are due to lack of time, resources and interruptions when performing this important administration of prescription only medicines. Vaccination clinic time should be protected and sufficient based on the number and type of vaccines to be given, the age and demographics of patients to be vaccinated and the person giving consent. If vaccinators are concerned that the time they have for a vaccination event is not safe for them or their patients, they are obliged to report this in writing to their management. Requests for more clinic time could be supported by the RCN Managing Childhood Immunisation Clinics (RCN, 2021), which recommends 20 min as the time required for best practice in child vaccination appointments.

10.5.3 Patient Arrival and Consultation

When the vaccine recipient and their carer arrive at the clinic, they should be met and greeted so that they feel welcomed and comfortable. The vaccinator should endeavour to convey to the vaccine recipient and carer that they are giving them their full attention, time is not an issue and they will devote their best efforts to providing a high-quality care experience.

Once settled, the vaccinator should check the vaccine recipient's knowledge of the vaccines to be offered; ideally when invited for vaccination, they should have been supplied with relevant leaflets or information. Although patients may have had some information before attending the clinic, it is still good practice for the vaccinator to inform the recipient or carer which vaccines are being offered that day and the diseases they are designed to protect against. Risks and benefits of vaccination should be outlined. Any common adverse events following vaccination should also be explained for each vaccine, before giving them. Although pre-clinic safety and eligibility checks may have been done, using medical records or consent forms, the vaccinator should make another check of the recipient's medical history, current health status, medications or treatments and any allergies. This final check, with the recipient present, will capture any recent changes that might not be recorded in the patient record or on any consent form. Any new information will inform further assessment of any potential contraindications, precautions and eligibility to a particular vaccine or vaccines.

An opportunity should be given for those being vaccinated, or giving consent for another, to ask any questions, obtain points of clarity and express concerns and worries if they have them. Maintaining the trust between patient and vaccinator is vital. If vaccinators cannot answer a patient's questions, they should acknowledge this and offer to find the information or ask a colleague who can assist. This offer should be followed through; the patient should not be left with unanswered questions. It is acknowledged that information and assurance from healthcare providers can be a decisive factor in parental decision about vaccine acceptance (Gust et al., 2008). All patients will benefit from the opportunity to talk to a well-educated vaccinator (Fig. 10.1).

Well-educated and trained vaccinators will gain confidence in answering patient queries over time but should also have the support of other more experienced colleagues if required. Additionally, they should ensure they remain up to date and/or have access to ongoing training and education.

Chapter 4 "Being a Safe Practitioner" covers more on this topic including education and skills competency requirements. Also see the Scope of Practice appendix.

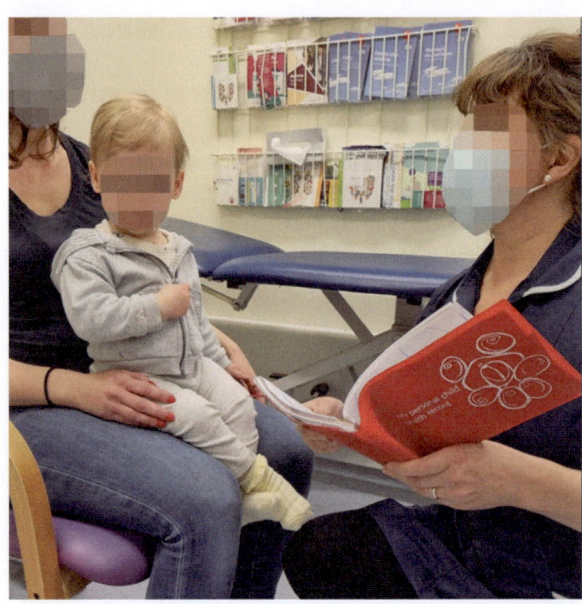

Fig. 10.1 Nurse discussing vaccination with a parent and child

10.5.4 Consent

When the patient or guardian has had the opportunity to have any questions answered, and the vaccinator is satisfied it is safe to offer the planned vaccines, the offer should be made, and consent obtained. The vaccinator should detail all aspects of the vaccination consultation including obtaining consent. Chapter 7 "Consent" covers consent in detail. If at any time the vaccinator is concerned that informed consent has not been obtained from a responsible and competent individual, then they should postpone vaccination until it has been obtained.

10.5.5 Addressing Vaccine Declines or Delay

As some parents/patients decline or delay vaccines, it is important that vaccinators are adept at handling the situation. The carer or recipient should be given the opportunity to explain their reasons for declining and, if necessary, be given a chance to ask further questions. The vaccinator should listen carefully to their rationale for declining and make an offer to discuss further. If the carer or recipient prefers not to discuss the matter further, the vaccinator should acknowledge this and advise that this will be noted in the clinical record. The risks of declining vaccines should be made clear to the patient or carer, giving details of the relevant vaccine preventable diseases, to which they remain susceptible. To support parents who may choose not to vaccinate their child, the risks and responsibilities of this decision could be discussed (WHO, 2017).

Vaccinators often worry about patients refusing vaccines for themselves or their children. The vaccinator's role is to ensure that potential vaccine recipients have all the information they need to reach an informed decision. Faced with refusal, the vaccinator needs to remain nonjudgemental, professional and accepting of their right to refuse. The vaccinator should make it clear that if the patient changes their mind and wishes to discuss vaccination in the future, they would be willing to discuss that with them. Chapter 6 "Discussing Vaccination with Patients" will give more guidance on managing vaccine refusal or delay.

10.5.6 Vaccine Preparation and Administration

Once consent has been obtained, vaccines should be prepared for administration. Vaccinators working to PGDs should not delegate any part of the vaccination process and should prepare and administer the vaccines themselves. In other settings, using other legal frameworks for delivering vaccines such as National Protocols, the process of preparing and giving vaccines may be split between several trained and competent healthcare workers. More on the preparation and administration of the vaccines is covered in Chap. 9 "Vaccine Administration".

10.5.7 Incidents and Errors

If it becomes apparent that an incident or error has occurred during or after the administration of vaccines, the vaccinator should remain calm, assess the situation and call for the assistance of colleagues if necessary. In most cases, reassurance can be given to the recipient or the carer that no immediate harm will come to the patient (RCN, 2021). The UKHSA "Vaccine incident guidance: responding to vaccine errors" provides invaluable guidance and information on responding to all types of errors in storage, handling and administration of vaccines (UKHSA, 2022). It is recommended that vaccinators familiarise themselves with this guidance and have timely access to it if needed. High-quality training and education will reduce errors but also enable vaccinators to respond appropriately should they happen. All errors should be reported, not only to the recipient but to the vaccination leads of the provider organisation, local commissioning immunisation team and Integrated Care Board. Vaccinators who make errors should ask for and embrace any subsequent investigation since establishing factors that led to error may result in better working arrangements for vaccinators, ensure higher levels of patient safety and inform best practice.

10.6   Following Vaccination

Prior to administering any vaccine, the vaccinator will have explained its purpose and any potential adverse events following vaccination and how to manage them. Many recipients can find the process of vaccination stressful, and this can result in poor retention of verbal information given at the time. The vaccine recipients should be given written information, instructions or links to relevant vaccination guidance to take away for future reference.

All vaccines should be supplied with a patient information leaflet (PIL) produced by the manufacturer, and this should be given to the patient. Copies of PILs can be downloaded from the Electronic Medicines Compendium website (https://www.medicines.org.uk/emc).

The UKHSA and the NHS produce publications and information to support discussions with vaccine recipients regarding what to expect after vaccination.

- What to expect after vaccination (information about the common side effects of vaccinations that might occur in babies and young children up to 5 years of age)—https://www.gov.uk/government/publications/what-to-expect-after-vaccinations
- What to expect after your COVID-19 vaccination—https://www.gov.uk/government/publications/covid-19-vaccination-what-to-expect-after-vaccination/what-to-expect-after-your-covid-19-vaccination
- MenB vaccine and paracetamol: information about the meningococcal B (MenB) vaccine and paracetamol use—https://www.gov.uk/government/publications/menb-vaccine-and-paracetamol
- NHS website: vaccinations—includes information about vaccination for all ages—https://www.nhs.uk/conditions/vaccinations/

10.7 Predeparture

On completion of the vaccination event, recipients and carers should be given any relevant information about future vaccination opportunities, when and to where they may be invited. This is also an opportunity for them to ask any further questions or clarify any information before leaving.

10.8 Postvaccination

10.8.1 Adverse Events Following Vaccination

Vaccinators should be familiar with the classifications of adverse effects following vaccination, which are detailed in the Green Book Chap. 8 "Vaccine Safety and Adverse Events Following Immunisation" (UKHSA, 2024).

Adverse events may fall into the following categories: programme-related, vaccine-induced, coincidental and unknown. Vaccinators should be familiar with the common adverse events that all patients might experience, as well as specific adverse events known to occur after certain vaccines or in certain types of patients. Summary of Product Characteristics sheets for each vaccine list common and rare adverse events noted to occur after administration. It is the vaccinator's responsibility to be aware of this information and able to discuss the common adverse events with vaccinees or their carers.

Common adverse events following the administration of many vaccines in the UK national programmes are pain and redness at the site of injection, achy muscles and joints, headache, malaise, fever and loss of appetite in younger recipients. These symptoms are primarily a manifestation of the immune response which the vaccines are intended to elicit. All vaccine recipients should be warned of the potential for these symptoms to occur post-vaccination and reassured this is a normal response. Information should be provided on self-care of these symptoms such as plenty of fluids, rest and appropriate doses of paracetamol or ibuprofen for discomfort or fever.

It is, of course, important to emphasise that if symptoms persist and are severe or they are unduly worried, they should seek medical advice by either seeing a healthcare professional or calling NHS 111.

Rare vaccine-induced adverse events have been identified following administration of some vaccines, and in some recipients, these include seizures, hypotonic-hyporesponsive episodes (HEE), idiopathic thrombocytopaenic purpura (ITP), acute arthropathy, allergic reactions and anaphylaxis.

Very rare adverse conditions can arise following administration of some vaccines, and the vaccinator should be willing and able to discuss these if recipients have concerns. UKHSA has information for healthcare professionals on vaccination rare side effects from the UKHSA GOV.UK Immunisation collection website.

Anaphylaxis following vaccination is rare compared to the rate observed for other classes of drugs and estimated to be <1–3 per million doses of vaccine (Bohlke et al., 2003; McNeil, 2019). Despite its rarity, onset can be rapid and life threatening, and consequently at every clinic and vaccination event, there must be an anaphylaxis kit available and a means of summoning help should an emergency occur. The Resuscitation Council UK recommend all clinical staff have annual basic life support and anaphylaxis update training.

During the COVID-19 vaccination programme, millions of doses of vaccine were administered, often by a workforce that had not previously been involved in vaccination services. Initially a high number of reports of anaphylaxis were made, but many of these were later confirmed not to be anaphylaxis. In response, the Resuscitation Council UK produced guidance for the management of anaphylaxis for vaccination settings from the Resuscitation Council UK website.

10.8.2 Observation Period

Due to the rarity of anaphylaxis, and other rapid onset adverse events following vaccination, there is no recommendation for vaccine recipients to be observed for a specific time following vaccination. However, a clinical decision may be made to observe the patient's condition for a time, for example, patients who have had a previous anaphylactic reaction to a related vaccine (as noted in the Green Book Chap. 14a for COVID-19 vaccines), but an observation period is not a routine requirement.

10.8.3 Adverse Event Reporting

Patients and carers should be reassured that the safety surveillance systems in place, following the introduction of new vaccines into the UK programme, work very efficiently; any safety signals are noted, and action taken if a vaccine needs to be withdrawn or restricted in its use.

If a vaccinator, vaccine recipient or their carer feels there has been an adverse event following vaccination, which was over and above what they would normally expect, this should be reported as part of the ongoing surveillance and monitoring mechanisms in place in the UK. The primary system for reporting adverse reactions to medicines, including vaccines, is the Yellow Card scheme managed by the MHRA. The MHRA also reports on the suspected side effects reported via the Yellow Card system.

Disease incidence is also reported by healthcare providers and laboratories to national surveillance systems. Such surveillance can reveal higher than background disease rates or expected levels of unusual or rare health conditions.

The Green Book Chap. 9 "Surveillance and Monitoring for Vaccine Safety" covers more detail on this topic.

Chapter 3 "Vaccine Development and Onward Management of Vaccine Safety" covers this in more detail.

10.9 Postvaccination Management

At the end of each vaccination event, the vaccinator should ensure all documentation is completed with all vaccination activity entered onto the patient record and/or national management systems. Each recording system will require the vaccinator to select the vaccine given, often requiring the selection of a code. Coding for vaccination, and the patient's underlying disease or condition (if appropriate), is important for identification of patients' eligibility for future vaccines, estimating vaccine uptake and coverage and, for some providers, payment purposes. Most systems will have text alongside the codes and multiple codes pertaining to the same vaccine; hence, careful selection is important. Many providers will be required to use nationally specified clinical coding in electronic health records (SNOMED codes), details of which can be found on the NHS Digital website (https://digital.nhs.uk/services/terminology-and-classifications/snomed-ct).

Additional administrative tasks will include noting patients who did not attend, declined or chose to delay the vaccination offer. It might be that patients will need following up, engagement with other healthcare providers (such has health visitors for children) or reappointing for a future vaccination offer.

If the vaccination event was the first of many, perhaps in a new venue or offering a new vaccine or to a new cohort, a post clinic wash-up meeting would be held to consider the strengths and weaknesses of the management arrangements and have the opportunity to make changes or improvements.

When vaccination activity has been captured, the vaccinator should complete the practical end of session tasks. Any unused vaccines, having been stored correctly, should be assessed for future use and returned to the fridge if safe to do so. Vaccines may need to be ordered for future clinics and sessions.

The venue should then be cleaned and prepared for future use. Waste should be disposed of in accordance with local waste management arrangements (see Chap. 11 "Infection Prevention and Control and Waste Management").

10.10 Conclusion

Public confidence in vaccines, and the national vaccination programmes, can be promoted by the provision of safe, efficient and easily accessible vaccination clinics, events and episodes.

The management of high-quality vaccination delivery, resulting in vaccine recipients who feel cared for and satisfied with their experience, requires knowledgeable leaders to make sound preparations and plans for delivery.

The other topics detailed in this book form the bedrock on which the sound management of vaccination clinics, events and episodes is built. Vaccinators need to be knowledgeable about the vaccine preventable diseases; the vaccines offered; what education, skills and competency they need to attain; and how to care for vaccines, communicate with patients and carers, adhere to legal requirements of consent and prescribing, correct vaccine administration and infection prevention and maximise uptake to promote both individual and population health.

All vaccinators can contribute to improving and promoting good clinic management, regardless of their position or grade in an organisation. The vaccination lead is key to ensure the organisation offers a successful, high-quality vaccination service. Each vaccinator, supported by other members of the vaccination team, can be a valuable contributor to that success.

References

Bohlke K, David RL, Marcy SH et al. (2003). Risk of anaphylaxis after vaccination of children and adolescents. *Pediatrics* **112**: 815–20. https://publications.aap.org/pediatrics/article-abstract/112/4/815/63454/Risk-of-Anaphylaxis-After-Vaccination-of-Children?redirectedFrom=fulltext

Dexter LJ, Teare MD, Dexter M, et al. (2012). Strategies to increase influenza vaccination rates: outcomes of a nationwide cross-sectional survey of UK general practice. *BMJ Open* http://bmjopen.bmj.com/content/2/3/e000851.full.pdf+html

Gust DA, Darling N, Kennedy A et al (2008). Parents With Doubts About Vaccines: Which Vaccines and Reasons Why. *Pediatrics*. **122**. (4). 718-725. https://publications.aap.org/pediatrics/article-abstract/122/4/718/71378/Parents-With-Doubts-About-Vaccines-Which-Vaccines

McNeil MM (2019). Vaccine-Associated Anaphylaxis. *Current Treatment Options Allergy*. **6**. (3): 297–308. https://www.ncbi.nlm.nih.gov/pmc/articles/PMC6896995/

Newby KV et al (2016). Identifying strategies to increase influenza vaccination in GP practices: a positive deviance approach. *Family Practice*. March; 1-6 http://fampra.

oxfordjournals.org/content/early/2016/03/28/fampra.cmw016.abstract?sid=c5869385-8624-44dc-92a1-e04aeda2192c

NICE guidance NG218 (2022). Vaccine uptake in the general population. https://www.nice.org.uk/guidance/ng218

Royal College of Nursing (RCN). (2021). Managing Childhood Immunisation Clinics. https://www.rcn.org.uk/Professional-Development/publications/managing-childhood-immunisation-clinics-uk-pub-009-860

Royal College of Nursing. (2022). Immunisation Knowledge and Skills Competence Assessment Tool. https://www.rcn.org.uk/professional-development/publications/immunisation-knowledge-and-skills-competence-assessment-tool-uk-pub-010-074

UK Health Security Agency (2022). Vaccine incident guidance: responding to vaccine errors. https://www.gov.uk/government/publications/vaccine-incident-guidance-responding-to-vaccine-errors

UK Health Security Agency (2024). Green Book - Immunisation against Infectious disease. https://www.gov.uk/government/collections/immunisation-against-infectious-disease-the-green-book

UKHSA (2025a). Guidance: Quality criteria for an effective immunisation programme https://www.gov.uk/government/publications/quality-criteria-for-an-effective-immunisation-programme (07/07/2025)

UKHSA (2025b). National Minimum Standards and Core Curriculum for Vaccination Training https://www.gov.uk/government/publications/national-minimum-standards-and-core-curriculum-for-immunisation-training-for-registered-healthcare-practitioners

WHO (2017). Information for parents. If you choose not to vaccinate your child, understand the risks and responsibilities. https://www.brookmedicalcentre.nhs.uk/wp-content/uploads/2020/06/If-you-choose_EN_WHO_WEB-1.pdf

Infection Prevention and Control Principles for Vaccination

11

Rose Gallagher

11.1 Introduction

The prevention of infection is a key element of quality health and care services and is applicable to vaccination regardless of the setting or situation in which they may be administered.

11.2 Maintaining the Quality of the Vaccine

Vaccine efficacy may be affected if storage conditions (too warm or too cold) or reconstitution practices are not optimal. This can result in inactivation of vaccines or reduced potency leading to reduced or no immunological response or protection against disease in those receiving vaccines. Vaccine storage is covered in detail in Chap. 5.

All staff administering vaccines should have received specific training on vaccination including the storage and reconstitution of vaccines in line with the "Green Book" *Immunisation Against Infectious Diseases* recommendations. Specific requirements for individual vaccines may be found in manufacturer's information and the Green Book (UKHSA online).

11.3 Protecting the Healthcare Workers

The protection of healthcare workers from infection in the workplace is reliant on several conditions being in place. Responsibility for safe systems of work is dependent on the healthcare worker (as an employee) and the employer meeting their

---

R. Gallagher (✉)
Royal College of Nursing, London, UK
e-mail: rose.gallagher@rcn.org.uk

© Springer Nature Switzerland AG 2025
H. Donovan, H. Bedford (eds.), *Safe Vaccine Administration*,
https://doi.org/10.1007/978-3-031-92498-9_11

legal and regulatory responsibilities for safety in the workplace. Employers have a legal duty to ensure, so far as is reasonably practicable, the health, safety and welfare at work of all their employees. Overarching legislation supporting this responsibility includes the Health and Safety at Work etc. Act 1974 and Health and Safety at Work Order (Northern Ireland). The Control of Substances Hazardous to Health (COSHH) (Health and Safety Executive online-a, online-b) and Health and Safety (Sharp Instruments in Healthcare) Regulations (Health and Safety Executive 2013) both support the prevention of infection. From a COSHH perspective, microorganisms such as bacteria and viruses capable of causing infection may be classified as biological hazards. This includes but is not limited to, for example, SARS-CoV-2 and hepatitis B and C. Actions supporting the prevention of infection include but are not limited to the need to provide and attend education and training sessions, ensuring optimal IPC practices are always implemented, the provision of personal protective equipment (PPE) and reporting of issues or concerns that may impact on the spread of infection.

11.3.1 Education and Meeting Local IPC Standards

All staff should receive education on infection prevention and control (IPC) when commencing employment and on a regular ongoing basis in line with employer's policies. Details on the specific requirements for frequency of education reflect individual countries' standards supporting IPC and typically range from annually to every 3 years as determined by the healthcare worker's role, responsibilities and workplace setting. This includes the Nursing and Midwifery Council expectations for registrants to keep knowledge and skills up to date through regular learning and professional development that maintains and develops an individual's competence (Nursing and Midwifery Council 2024). This is in addition to vaccine training, and all staff should be familiar and comply with their local IPC policies and procedures.

When considering the protection of healthcare workers, both proactive and reactive measures will be implemented at different times. The wellbeing and safety of staff requires the collaboration and support of occupational health services, health and safety teams, infection prevention and control teams/advisors and managers as well as individual health and care professionals. Specific expectations for the prevention of infection can be found in national standards and guidance. These set out what is required to enable an organisational culture whereby infection prevention and control is a core domain of the delivery of safe and effective care. Examples can be found in NICE guidance (2014) and national IPC standards such as Infection Prevention and Control Standards (Health Improvement Scotland 2022), Health and Social Care Act 2008: Code of Practice on the Prevention and Control of Infections (Department of Health and Social Care 2022), Code of Practice for the Prevention and Control of Healthcare Associated Infections (Welsh Government 2014).

11.4 Best Practice for Prevention of Infection with Vaccine Administration

Standard precautions underpin the protection of both the healthcare worker and vaccine recipient from potential transmission of infection.

They include the most common practices such as hand hygiene, safe disposal of sharps/waste and cleanliness of the environment.

The following should be considered as integral elements relevant to vaccination practice:

- Storage, preparation and administration of vaccines and associated equipment (Chap. 5)
- Hand hygiene and skin integrity
- Use of personal protective equipment (PPE)
- Disposal of waste/sharps
- Environmental cleanliness
- Transmission of infection between staff
- Reporting of incidents

11.4.1 Hand Hygiene

Hand hygiene is effective in preventing the transmission of microbes (e.g. bacteria and viruses) between people through direct contact. It can be achieved using soap and water as part of hand washing or the use of alcohol-based hand sanitisers. Spread of microbes via hands can occur following direct contact between people and the environment. The fundamental principles of good hand hygiene include the following:

- Always cleaning hands before preparing vaccines and direct contact with patients. To enhance patient/person trust, this is ideally undertaken in front of patients.
- Not wearing stoned rings or wrist watches/bracelets while at work. A plain wedding band is acceptable. This ensures hands can be cleaned effectively and harm, such as scratches, do not occur through contact with staff jewellery. A professional image also helps instil public and patient confidence.
- Use a hand hygiene technique in line with local policies/training.

For hand hygiene to be effective, the following is required:

- Provision of correct equipment (alcohol hand sanitizer, soap and running water, single use hand towels). Where mobile vaccination clinics are in place, portable hand washing basins are acceptable provided clean water is available. Shared cloth hand towels are not acceptable.
- Intact skin on hands/wrists.

Skin health is essential for wellbeing of the individual member of staff and the ability to undertake effective hand hygiene.

11.4.2 Skin Health

The main function of the skin is protection of internal tissues and organs. It is the largest organ of the body and acts as a barrier to prevent fluid loss, preventing microorganisms from entering the body, and to modify the effects of pressure, radiation, heat, chemicals and trauma on internal body systems. If the skin is disrupted or damaged, it cannot undertake this function effectively (Royal College of Nursing 2022).

Dermatitis is common among nurses (Royal College of Nursing 2020) with an estimated 1000 healthcare workers developing work-related contact dermatitis a year (Health and Safety Executive—Dermatitis in health care online). The true scale of work-related dermatitis however is likely to be much greater as national surveillance systems to monitor its prevalence are not in place.

Symptoms of dermatitis range from mild to severe. The most common symptoms include redness, itching, cracked skin/weeping/bleeding and thickening of the skin. People experiencing these symptoms are unlikely to be able to undertake hand hygiene as exposure to soap and water or alcohol hand sanitiser will be painful and exacerbate symptoms. This situation may require staff being moved to non-clinical/patient contact duties until symptoms are resolved.

More information can be found in the RCN (2022) guidance. To support effective hand hygiene and prevent dermatitis or manage in a timely way, the following should be in place:

- Regular skin checks and immediate reporting of any symptoms identified to enable assessment and any treatment to commence as soon as possible.
- Adoption of a three-step approach to dermatitis—avoid, protect, check by employers (RCN 2022)
- Clear policies on the use of gloves to reduce excessive glove use when not required (see use of personal protective equipment)
- The provision of hand cream/hand emollients in the workplace

11.4.3 Use of Personal Protective Equipment (PPE)

PPE is required to protect healthcare professionals from hazards in the workplace. Hands may be exposed to potential hazards in healthcare such as biological hazards (microbes capable of causing infection) and harmful drugs or chemicals (including environmental disinfectants).

PPE should be used where exposure to the known or potential harm cannot be removed or managed in other ways. Gloves are frequently used in healthcare settings as exposure to blood and body fluids is a common hazard. Wearing gloves frequently or for long periods of time is a known cause of overhydration of the skin on hands potentially leading to dermatitis. Gloves are not recommended, therefore, where there is minimal or no risk present. In these situations, good hand hygiene is sufficient to maintain safe clinical practice.

Vaccination is generally considered a low-risk practice, and gloves *are not* routinely required for vaccine preparation and administration (WHO 2021; Royal College of Nursing 2021). Gloves may be worn when preparing BCG vaccine.

Aprons are rarely required in vaccination clinics, and avoiding unnecessary use is a positive way to reduce the unnecessary use of plastic in healthcare services, a key priority of sustainability strategies, for consumables derived from fossil fuels.

11.4.4 Disposal of Waste/Sharps

Health and care services produce a significant amount of waste. This includes sharps and pharmaceutical waste. Guidance such as Health Technical Memorandum 07-01 (NHS England 2022) outlines how waste should be managed aligned to national waste legislation, with sharps management specifically included within the Health and Safety (Sharp Instruments in Healthcare) Regulations 2013.

Sharps injuries frequently occur in healthcare and carry the risk of acquiring blood borne diseases such as hepatitis B and C and HIV if the sharp has been used for a patient with an infection. The impact on individuals exposed to such risks following a high-risk sharps injury is significant. More information can be found in RCN guidance "Sharps Safety" (Royal College of Nursing 2023).

The following best practice points support the prevention of infection:

- Sharps containers must be available at the point of use to prevent staff from carrying used sharps, avoiding unintentional "stabbing" injuries.
- Safer sharps devices should be used if available, and where used staff must be trained in their use.
- All sharps injuries should be reported, including "clean" injuries where the sharps has not been used on a patient. This enables data to be collected on how injuries occur to facilitate learning to prevent sharps injuries from occurring.
- Needles should never be re-sheathed; the entire "unit" of syringe and needle should be disposed of into a sharps container immediately following use.
- Sharps containers should be closed and sealed once the "fill line" is reached. This avoids overfilling and potential sharps injuries caused by contact with sharps bins.

The management of sharps as a waste category is described within Health Technical Memorandum 07-01 (NHS England 2022). Sustainable options to reduce the carbon footprint of healthcare waste include the use of reusable sharps bins which are cleaned after use avoiding incineration of single plastic sharps containers (Royal College of Nursing 2022). This option may be available to vaccination services, and advice should be sought from waste managers on local options available.

11.4.5 Other Waste

Most waste produced because of vaccination will be municipal (household) or offensive waste—minimal waste classified as infectious clinical waste will be produced. Health Technical Memorandum 07-01 (NHS England 2022) provides more detail on waste classification.

Waste is costly to dispose of and is a significant contributor to health services carbon footprint. National (NHS England 2023) and local waste strategies will provide more information on how to reduce the costs and improve sustainability associated with waste management including recycling where available.

11.4.6 Environmental Cleanliness

It is important to consider whether environment where care or services are delivered may be a potential reservoir of harmful microbes. The risk of harm and transfer of microbes between the environment and susceptible patients varies depending on the level of risk present. For example, intensive care units and operating theatres would be considered high-risk areas, while public areas and vaccination clinics are generally considered low risk as patients/people are dressed usually well (to receive vaccination) and no invasive procedures are undertaken.

Cleaning of the environment and cleanliness of equipment are still important in vaccination clinics; however, the widespread use of chemical disinfectants is not required. Likewise, vaccination in people's own homes/care homes does not require any specific additional measures beyond standard IPC precautions.

Local policies will provide information on cleaning schedules in clinics and responsibility for environmental cleaning tasks. Any member of staff whose role includes cleaning must have been trained on how to clean and the use of cleaning products. Regular cleanliness audits will support monitoring of the environment to ensure staff and patient confidence.

11.4.7 Preventing the Spread of Infection Between Staff

Staff should be mindful of the potential for staff-to-staff transmission of infection when sharing a work environment including communal staff areas such as offices and staff rooms. Infections such as, but not limited to, norovirus and respiratory illnesses (colds, influenza, RSV and COVID-19) are easily spread from person to person. Staff should not work if they are unwell due to the risk of transmitting infection to other staff or patients/public and refer to local policies for more information on reporting and management of sickness absence.

Note: Learning on the value and use of ventilation is currently ongoing at the time of publication to support the prevention of transmission of infection from person to person via the respiratory route in enclosed environments such as clinics, wards, etc.

11.5 Summary

Prevention of infection is a key requirement for ensuring safety and quality in all health and care services. Vaccination is a relatively low-risk procedure, but the principles of good infection prevention and control must be adhered to, regardless of the setting or situation where it is being caried out. This is essential to ensure vaccine efficacy as outlined in Chap. 5 and to make sure patients and staff are protected as far as possible from infection as a result of the procedure.

References

Department of Health and Social Care (2022). Health and Social Care Act 2008: code of practice on the prevention and control of infections https://www.gov.uk/government/publications/the-health-and-social-care-act-2008-code-of-practice-on-the-prevention-and-control-of-infections-and-related-guidance

Health and Safety Executive (online-a). Control of substances hazardous to health regulations 2002 (as amended in 2004) - General enforcement guidance and advice OC273/20 https://www.hse.gov.uk/foi/internalops/ocs/200-299/273_20/#Regulation-6 [Accessed October 2024]

Health and Safety Executive (2013) Health and Safety (Sharp Instruments in Healthcare) Regulations 2013 https://www.hse.gov.uk/pubns/hsis7.htm [Accessed October 2024]

Health and Safety Executive (online-b). Dermatitis in health and social care https://www.hse.gov.uk/healthservices/dermatitis.htm#:~:text=Each%20year%20an%20estimated%201000,%2C%20redness%2C%20cracking%20and%20blistering. [Accessed October 2024]

Health Improvement Scotland (2022). Healthcare Associated Infection (HAI) standards https://www.healthcareimprovementscotland.org/our_work/standards_and_guidelines/stnds/hai_standards_2015.aspx [Accessed October 2024]

NHS England (2022). Health Technical Memorandum 07-01: Safe and sustainable management of healthcare waste https://www.england.nhs.uk/wp-content/uploads/2021/05/B2159iii-health-technical-memorandum-07-01.pdf [Accessed October 2024]

NHS England (2023). NHS clinical waste strategy NHS England » NHS clinical waste strategy [Accessed October 2024]

National Institute for Health and Care Excellence (2014) Infection prevention and control. Quality standard [QS61] https://www.nice.org.uk/guidance/qs61 [Accessed October 2024]

Nursing and Midwifery Council (2024) 'The Code' https://www.nmc.org.uk/standards/code/

Welsh Government (2014). Code of Practice for the Prevention and Control of Healthcare Associated Infections https://www.gov.wales/sites/default/files/publications/2019-06/code-of-practice-for-the-prevention-and-control-of-healthcare-associated-infections.pdf

Royal College of Nursing (2020) RCN Survey exploring skin health issues among nursing staff in the UK: results of a national survey. A project commissioned by the Royal College of Nursing Via RCN Learn https://www.rcn.org.uk/

Royal College of Nursing (2021). Why you don't always need gloves when giving vaccines https://www.rcn.org.uk/magazines/Clinical/2021/July/Why-you-dont-always-need-gloves-when-giving-vaccines-COVID-19

Royal College of Nursing (2022) Tools of the Trade https://www.rcn.org.uk/Professional-Development/publications/tools-of-the-trade-uk-pub-010-218

Royal College of Nursing (2023). Sharps safety https://www.rcn.org.uk/Professional-Development/publications/rcn-sharps-safety-uk-pub-010-596

UKHSA (online). Immunisation against infectious disease, the 'Green Book' https://www.gov.uk/government/collections/immunisation-against-infectiousdisease-the-green-book

WHO (2021). Infection prevention and control (IPC) principles and procedures for COVID-19 vaccination activities. https://iris.who.int/bitstream/handle/10665/338715/WHO-2019-nCoV-vaccination-IPC-2021.1-eng.pdf

Maximising Vaccine Uptake: A Population/Community Approach

12

Louise Letley

12.1 Introduction

Despite a gradual decline in childhood vaccination uptake since 2013/14 (ref), vaccine confidence generally remains high. Improving immunisation coverage rates across the UK. https://www.bma.org.uk/what-we-do/population-health/improving-care-and-peoples-experience-ofservices/improving-immunisation-coverage-rates-across-the-uk. Surveys of parents of infants in England have been carried out for over 30 years. Since 2015, annual surveys have consistently shown a high level of confidence in the routine vaccine programme in the UK (Campbell et al. 2017, 2023). The 2023 survey found that over 80% of parents agreed that vaccines work and that they are safe (UKHSA 2023a). However, a Public Health England health equity audit of the national immunisation programme (PHE 2017) found that inequalities existed within certain population groups including underserved communities such as travellers, migrants, prisoners and looked-after children.

Immunisation is one of the most cost-effective public health interventions with childhood immunisation in particular enabling children to thrive and get the best start in life. It is estimated that immunisation prevents between three and five million deaths from vaccine preventable diseases annually worldwide (WHO online). As such, striving for equality in vaccine uptake is an important way to address health inequalities. Ensuring that coverage is also high within underserved communities is essential both for individuals and for disease control and elimination strategies. This chapter will explore the importance of reducing inequalities in immunisation and adapting immunisation programmes to meet the needs of local populations.

L. Letley (✉)
UK Health Security Agency (UKHSA), London, UK
e-mail: Louise.letley@ukhsa.gov.uk

© Springer Nature Switzerland AG 2025
H. Donovan, H. Bedford (eds.), *Safe Vaccine Administration*,
https://doi.org/10.1007/978-3-031-92498-9_12

12.2 Health Inequalities

The King's Fund states that "health inequalities mean that some population groups have significantly worse health outcomes and experiences than others. These inequalities are avoidable, unfair and systematic" (Kings Fund 2022). The United Nations has set reducing inequalities within and between countries as one of the Sustainable Development Goals (SDGs). The 17 SDGs were adopted by all UN Member States in 2015, as part of the 2030 Agenda for Sustainable Development which set out a 15-year plan to achieve the Goals (United Nations online).

Health professionals have a duty to reduce inequalities, e.g. in England, there is a requirement under the Public Sector Equality Duty section of the Equality Act 2010 (UK Gov 2010) for all public authorities to promote equality of opportunity, preventing discrimination, harassment and victimisation and fostering good relations between the different protected characteristics groups. Additionally, under the Health and Social Care Act 2012 (UK Gov 2012), the NHS has a legal duty to offer immunisation to "hard to reach groups, for example gypsy traveller children or looked-after children, who may require special and specific arrangements" and people "moving into the country from abroad who have incomplete or unknown vaccination status". In the UK devolved administrations, there are similar requirements as part of a fundamental human right.

12.3 Know Your Community

As ensuring individuals, particularly young children, are up to date with their vaccinations is an effective way of reducing health inequalities, it is important for all immunisers to be aware of the specific needs of their population and any barriers to vaccination.

Asking Specifically
- Are there any specific groups within your community that may have unmet needs?
- Do the services provided meet the needs of these communities, or can they be tailored to reduce inequalities?

Recent NICE guidance (NICE 2022) highlighted some population groups that are known to have low vaccine uptake or be at risk of low uptake (see Box 12.1). Health professionals have a duty to ensure that everyone who is eligible for immunisation is offered and that services provided are accessible to all.

> **Box 12.1 Population Groups That Are Known to have Low Vaccine Uptake or Be At Risk of Low Uptake**
> - People from some minority ethnic family backgrounds
> - People from Gypsy, Roma and Traveller communities
> - People with physical or learning disabilities
> - People from some religious communities (e.g. Orthodox Jewish)
> - New migrants and asylum seekers
> - Looked-after children and young people
> - Children of young or lone parents
> - Children from large families
> - People who live in an area of high deprivation
> - Babies or children who are hospitalised or have a chronic illness and their siblings
> - People not registered with a GP
> - People from non-English-speaking families
> - People who are homeless

12.4 Using Data to Identify Underserved Communities

Good data is key and can help identify population groups with suboptimal vaccine uptake. It is essential for immunisers to become familiar with the demographics of the community and population they are responsible for alongside the vaccine uptake. There are many sources of data that provide information on national and local populations including demographic statistics from census data, government and local government reports and health data. Vaccination uptake data is widely available at local level, and it is also relatively straightforward to set up tailored searches on most electronic health systems that can be saved and run as required.

National coverage reports and data tables are also available online providing snapshots of quarterly and annual uptake data broken down by local government areas, for example, in England, there is an interactive dashboard that enables comparison of vaccination uptake across local government areas for the routine childhood programme up to 5 years of age (NHS Digital online) and a public health database that enables searching across indicators such as deprivation (OHID online)

12.5 Recording Vaccination Data

To ensure that both local and national data outputs and reports are as accurate as possible, it is important to ensure timely and accurate recording of all vaccinations given. Search results on any computer system are only as good as the data entered, so consideration should be made whether there are any improvements that could be made to local data collection systems to ensure easy identification of who is due for vaccines. For example, consider recording details such as ethnicity and whether individuals are non-English speakers/readers or are members of a specific underserved community, so they can be added to bespoke searches. This will enable accurate, timely and appropriate invitation and reminders to be sent out and followed up if there is no response, the "call and recall" systems.

If any vaccinations take place outside the usual settings, for example, in schools, it is imperative that there is a clear pathway for details to reach individual health records and that everyone involved in the process is aware of their responsibilities. Ensuring the individual's health record is complete enables opportunities to offer and advise on vaccines missed during school or other vaccination settings.

12.6 Reducing Inequalities

Once communities or groups with unmet needs have been identified, consideration should be given to what additional support could be provided to reduce inequalities in vaccination uptake. This includes checking with local stakeholders and searching for available evidence on strategies/interventions that have been tested in similar populations and any recommendations for tailoring services. It is worth bearing in mind that there are differences between and within underserved groups and as such there is no "one size fits all" strategy, so multiple approaches may be necessary, for example, methods of communication and how services are delivered may need to be adapted.

12.7 Local Knowledge

There may be valuable insights about underserved communities to be gained from other local stakeholders including those in the health and social care, education, local government and third sector organisations. Community support organisations often provide reports highlighting issues and recommendations for working with their specific communities.

12.8 Available Evidence

In addition to national and local data sources, there is also some published evidence on underserved communities and their experiences of the routine vaccination programme. The results highlight that issues with accessing services are common and suggest ways on how to work with communities to improve uptake. Three case studies are detailed below.

Case Study 12.1: Charedi Orthodox Jewish community in Hackney
The London borough of Hackney is home to one of the largest Charedi Orthodox Jewish communities, outside Israel and New York. The Charedi community was already established in Stamford Hill in the 1920s, but the population increased significantly during the Second World War as new arrivals fled the Holocaust. Membership of the community is not systematically recorded in medical records but is estimated at around 30,000. Immunisation uptake within the community is consistently lower than the rest of the borough and the rest of England. Suboptimal immunisation coverage has led to recurrent outbreaks of vaccine preventable diseases.

In 2015, PHE and NHS England in collaboration with WHO Europe used the "Tailoring Immunisation Programmes" (TIP) approach with the Charedi community (Letley et al. 2018). TIP was developed by WHO Europe to identify susceptible populations, determine barriers to vaccination and implement evidence-based interventions. Community members and religious leaders were involved at all stages of the project and were key to its success.

There was no evidence of religious or community-wide anti-vaccination beliefs. Families within the community were of larger than average size, so many of the issues related to access and convenience of immunisation services. Service providers in the area had challenges due to having to provide call and recall and deliver immunisation services to the large numbers of children without additional resource. Where mothers were choosing to delay or decline vaccinations, their reasons were broadly similar to the wider population. Other issues identified included lack of up-to-date community specific communications, a need for improved recording of community membership and evaluation of any community specific interventions.

Case Study 12.2: Traveller Communities
Most travellers in England are Irish Travellers, Gypsies or Roma. The Irish Traveller community is categorised as an ethnic minority group under the Race Relations Act 1976 (amended 2000), the Human Rights Act 1998 and the Equality Act 2010. In the 2021 census (ONS 2022), almost 68,000 people identified as "Gypsy or Irish Traveller", and over 100,000 people identified as "Roma". This is likely to be a large underestimate as other statistics such as biannual Traveller caravan count and school roll figures suggest that there are probably more like 200,000–300,000 Romany Gypsy and Traveller people living in England and Wales (Travellers Times 2022). It is widely accepted that Travellers, Gypsies and Roma have some of the worst outcomes for a wide range of social indicators including health when compared to other communities. Membership of traveller communities is not consistently recorded

(continued)

or monitored by the NHS; therefore, assessing immunisation uptake and developing services to meet community needs can be challenging.

In 2015, an immunisation audit (Dixon et al. 2017) in a General Practice in the East of England serving a high proportion of Irish Travellers found that only 45% of Irish Traveller children had two MMR doses by 5 years of age compared to 90% of non-Traveller children. This General Practice had a good relationship with the local Traveller population, and so coverage elsewhere could be even lower.

The UNITING study team (Jackson et al. 2016) carried out an interview study with Travellers and service providers followed by workshops to identify priorities. The study identified good examples of specialist immunisation services, but these were not universally available. The study confirmed that most Travellers are pro-vaccine and that most concerns and access issues were similar to those of the wider population. There were some community specific issues such as feeling judged unfavourably by some health professionals because of their lifestyle.

The UNITING study participants identified and prioritised five interventions to improve immunisation uptake:

1. Cultural competence training for health professionals and frontline staff
2. Identification of Travellers in health records to tailor support and monitor uptake
3. Provision of a named frontline person in General Practices to provide a respectful and supportive service
4. Flexible and diverse systems for booking appointments, recall and reminders
5. Protected funding for health visitors specialising in Traveller health, including immunisation

Case Study 12.3: Migrant Populations
When the European Union expanded in 2004 and 2007, there was an increase in the Eastern European born population in the UK. In 2021, it was estimated that there were almost 700,000 Polish and 342,000 Romanian residents living in the UK (ONS 2021). Despite differences in vaccination schedules, vaccination coverage and vaccine confidence between countries, there was little work to highlight the unmet needs of the community.

In 2019, the results of a qualitative study (Bell et al. 2019) focusing on vaccine-related attitudes and behaviours among Polish and Romanian communities in England were published. In-depth semi structured interviews with Polish and Romanian community members and healthcare workers (HCWs)

(continued)

involved in the provision and delivery of vaccinations in areas with high Polish and Romanian populations had been carried out.

Although most community members reported accepting vaccination and vaccinating according to the UK schedule, some experienced difficulties navigating and trusting the English primary healthcare system. This was partly due to differences in vaccination scheduling and service provision in England, such as nurses delivering vaccines instead of doctors and babies not getting a check-up by a doctor prior to vaccination. Challenges in accessing credible vaccination information in Polish and Romanian were also reported. Others continued to get their children vaccinated in Poland on trips to visit family.

The authors made a series of recommendations for tailoring services for the Polish and Romanian communities. They emphasised that HCWs should discuss health service expectations, highlight differences in vaccination scheduling and delivery between countries and promote greater understanding of the English primary healthcare system.

12.9 Suggestions for Working with Underserved Communities

Based on some of this evidence, the following are some suggestions for improving uptake.

Community/cultural awareness training: some communities offer this training to staff involved in healthcare to give them a better understanding of their cultures, traditions and histories. It can also provide insight into the barriers they face when accessing services and how HCWs can support them better, e.g. Friends, Families and Travellers (English national charity working with and on behalf of the Gypsy, Roma and Traveller communities) provide a digital cultural awareness training package (Friends, Families and Travellers online).

Community engagement and advocacy: Community involvement was highlighted as key in the three case histories detailed above.
- Some service providers have successfully worked with religious leaders or other individuals respected within the community to promote immunisation.
- Some areas are taking engagement a step further by localising vaccination services. During the COVID-19 pandemic, commissioners and providers of the vaccination programme worked with Hatzola, a volunteer emergency service providing services to the Charedi (sometimes referred to as Haredi) Jewish community in London. Hatzola hosted vaccination sessions and was responsible for promotion of the programme, distributing appointments and administering vaccines. A qualitative study (Kasstan et al. 2022) exploring the views of those involved in the collaboration concluded that "Localising vac-

cination services raises opportunities for greater vaccine equity by supporting ethnic and religious minorities to collaborate in safeguarding community health and wellbeing".
- Some communities have support organisations who may be prepared to advise on communications or the design of other proposed interventions.

Accessibility of services: A recurring theme in research into underserved communities.

What improvements could be made to immunisation services to increase flexibility and inclusiveness? Some of this is also considered in Chap. 10 but worth further thought here in relation to maximising vaccine uptake.
- Consider the venue. Are the current services held in a place that is easy to get to without too much time or expense?
- Do the timings of clinics work for those using public transport?
- Is it worth considering other venues for vulnerable groups, for example, a familiar place within their own community such as a community or children's centre or even targeted home visits? These may be more expensive to deliver, but incident response and outbreak management, in addition to the impact on affected individuals, are extremely resource intensive and expensive. An economic evaluation showed that a measles outbreak in 2012–2013 in Merseyside costs more than 20 times the cost of the vaccinations that could have prevented it (Ghebrehewet et al. 2016).
- Are the facilities, services and staff welcoming? It is an adage but "you never get a second chance to make a first impression".
- Do all levels of staff recognise the importance of being inclusive? Lack of identification, proof of address or immigration status should not be a barrier to registration or immunisation.
- Do staff introduce themselves and explain processes?
- Consider whether waiting areas are appropriate. Is there enough room for prams? Is there a space for breastfeeding women who require privacy to do so?
- Is there enough flexibility within the appointment system for those who can't turn up on a specific day or time or have unpredictable lives?
- Are there a variety of appointment options, different days of the week, times of the day and drop-in? Is there room for opportunistic vaccination within the service, e.g. if a child who is due for vaccination attends the service with another family member, could they be vaccinated there and then?
- Timing: Are appointment times long enough? Underserved communities may have additional needs with regard to language and literacy and shouldn't feel hurried. It is important that they have a chance to ask questions so that they can be comfortable with their decisions. Additionally, if appointment times are too short, then waiting times can increase leading to dissatisfaction with services.

Communications: Are communications relevant and appropriate?

HCPs are an extremely important and trusted source of vaccination information and so have a very important role in supporting people in their vaccine decisions. The figure for HCP and NHS trust is that over 80% of parents ranked health care

professionals and the NHS in their top three most trusted sources for vaccination information (UKHSA 2023a). Following a discussion with an HCP 66% of parents felt more confident about having their child vaccinated and 14% who had not made up their minds, decided to vaccinate (UKHSA 2023a).
- A phone call a few days before an appointment (especially for the first immunisation appointment of the infant schedule) to introduce yourself and answer any questions may make the parents more comfortable on the day. Let them know what is involved in the vaccination appointment, and ensure they are aware that vaccination services are free in the UK.
  – Have people with different language and literacy needs been considered? Requirements should be determined at the time of registering for services. These should be recorded so prior arrangements can be put in place to avoid unnecessary barriers to immunisation discussions and consent.
- Do people understand that the vaccination offer generally remains ongoing even when appointments have been missed? For most vaccines, it is never too late to catch up.
  – Written information: Are there versions in different languages available? For example, in England, the UKHSA provides information leaflets for the routine immunisation programme in multiple languages, easy read, braille, video and audio. They are produced at national level and are available free of charge. Most are also available to order in hard copy for those who haven't got access to digital services (Health Publications online).
  – Verbal communication: Are parents given an opportunity to discuss vaccination and have their questions answered with a healthcare professional (HCP), ideally before the vaccination appointment? Interpretation services, where a conversation or discussion is reproduced in another language, may be required for some populations where English is not their first language. Services are usually commissioned locally and should be free at the point of delivery for the patient. It is best practice not to use a relative or friend to interpret to maintain patient confidentiality.

12.10 Intervention and Evaluation

It is important to ensure that any new intervention to improve vaccine uptake is appropriately designed and evaluated to ensure effectiveness, sustainability and value for money (value doesn't necessarily mean cheaper). Tailoring immunisation programmes (WHO 2019) provides step by step guidance to identify suboptimally vaccinated populations, determine barriers and drivers and design interventions. An evaluation framework tool and guidance including explanatory video clips are also available online (UKHSA 2023b). The evaluation framework tool was produced to help with designing and implementing immunisation and vaccination interventions. It aims to be accessible to those who have not evaluated interventions before, as well as those who are more experienced. Although the designing, intervention and evaluation process undoubtedly requires significant time and effort, the framework tool helps users focus on modifiable factors and reduces duplication by prepopulating subsequent documents with previously entered relevant information.

The framework uses the capability, opportunity, motivation, behaviour (COM-B) model to help identify drivers and barriers to immunisation uptake to feed into the intervention design. It then automatically produces a figure based on the identified drivers and barriers to help inform the design of the intervention. Once an intervention has been identified and described, the tool produces a logic model figure to feed into the development of the evaluation guiding the user through each stage.

12.11 Summary

HCPs can reduce inequalities in vaccine services by identifying underserved communities within their population. By working with these communities to identify barriers and drivers to vaccination, solutions can be found so that services meet the needs of all members of society.

References

Bell S, Edelstein M, Zatoński M, Ramsay M, Mounier-Jack S. 'I don't think anybody explained to me how it works': qualitative study exploring vaccination and primary health service access and uptake amongst Polish and Romanian communities in England. BMJ Open. 2019 Jul 9;9(7):e028228. https://doi.org/10.1136/bmjopen-2018-028228. PMID: 31289079; PMCID: PMC6615777.

Campbell H, Edwards A, Letley L, Bedford H, Ramsay M, Yarwood J. Changing attitudes to childhood immunisation in English parents. Vaccine. 2017 May 19;35(22):2979–2985. https://doi.org/10.1016/j.vaccine.2017.03.089. Epub 2017 Apr 23. PMID: 28442229.

Campbell HP. Paterson L. Letley V. Saliba S. Mounier-Jack J. Yarwood, Vaccination, information and parental confidence in the digital age in England, Vaccine: X, Volume 14, 2023, 100345, ISSN 2590-1362

Dixon KC, Mullis R, Blumenfeld T. Vaccine uptake in the Irish Travelling community: an audit of general practice records. J Public Health (Oxf). 2017 Dec 1;39(4):e235–e241. https://doi.org/10.1093/pubmed/fdw088. PMID: 27642124.

Friends, Families and Travellers (online): Training Packages - Friends, Families and Travellers (gypsy-traveller.org)

Ghebrehewet S, Thorrington D, Farmer S, et al. The economic cost of measles: Healthcare, public health and societal costs of the 2012–13 outbreak in Merseyside, UK. Vaccine. 2016;34(15):1823–31.

Health Publications (online): http://www.healthpublications.gov.uk/Home.html

Jackson C, Dyson L, Bedford H, Cheater FM, Condon L, Crocker A, Emslie C, Ireland L, Kemsley P, Kerr S, Lewis HJ, Mytton J, Overend K, Redsell S, Richardson Z, Shepherd C, Smith L. UNderstanding uptake of Immunisations in TravellIng aNd Gypsy communities (UNITING): a qualitative interview study. Health Technol Assess. 2016 Sep;20(72):1–176. https://doi.org/10.3310/hta20720. PMID: 27686875; PMCID: PMC5056337.PMCID: PMC4466610.

Kasstan B, Mounier-Jack S, Letley L, Gaskell KM, Roberts CH, Stone NRH, Lal S, Eggo RM, Marks M, Chantler T. Localising vaccination services: Qualitative insights on public health and minority group collaborations to co-deliver coronavirus vaccines. Vaccine. 2022 Mar 25;40(14):2226–2232. https://doi.org/10.1016/j.vaccine.2022.02.056. Epub 2022 Feb 17. PMID: 35216844; PMCID: PMC8849863.

Kings Fund (2022): What are health inequalities. What Are Health Inequalities? | The King's Fund (kingsfund.org.uk)

Letley L, Rew V, Ahmed R, Habersaat KB, Paterson P, Chantler T, Saavedra-Campos M, Butler R. Tailoring immunisation programmes: Using behavioural insights to identify barriers and enablers to childhood immunisations in a Jewish community in London, UK. Vaccine. 2018 Jul 25;36(31):4687–4692. https://doi.org/10.1016/j.vaccine.2018.06.028. Epub 2018 Jun 23. PMID: 29945834.

NHS Digital (online): Childhood Vaccination Coverage Statistics- England, 2021-22 http://digital.nhs.uk/data-and-information/publications/statistical/nhs-immunisation-statistics/2021-22#resources

NICE: Vaccine uptake in the general population. London: National Institute for Health and Care Excellence (NICE); 2022 May 17. (NICE Guideline, No. 218.) Available from: http://www.ncbi.nlm.nih.gov/books/NBK581883/

OHID (online): Health Protection Profile covering a range of health protection issues, including immunisation http://fingertips.phe.org.uk/profile/health-protection/data#page/0/gid/1938132804/pat/6/par/E12000004/ati/102/are/E06000015

ONS 2021: Population of the UK by country of birth and nationality: year ending June 2021 http://www.ons.gov.uk/peoplepopulationandcommunity/populationandmigration/internationalmigration/bulletins/ukpopulationbycountryofbirthandnationality/yearendingjune2021#non-uk-populations-analysis

ONS 2022: Census Ethnicity Data https://www.ons.gov.uk/peoplepopulationandcommunity/culturalidentity/ethnicity/bulletins/ethnicgroupenglandandwales/census2021

Travellers Times (2022): Other GRT estimates http://www.travellerstimes.org.uk/news/2022/11/england-and-wales-census-2021-results-released-roma-included-first-ever-time#:~:text=67%2C768%20people%20identified%20as%20'Gypsy,time%20this%20category%20was%20included.

UK Government: Equality Act 2010 http://www.legislation.gov.uk/ukpga/2010/15/contents

UK Government: Health and Social Care Act 2012 http://www.legislation.gov.uk/ukpga/2012/7/contents/enacted

UKHSA 2023a Childhood vaccines: parental attitudes survey 2023 findings https://www.gov.uk/government/publications/childhood-vaccines-parental-attitudes-survey-2023/childhood-vaccinesparental-attitudes-survey-2023-findings#:~:text=Vaccine%20safety,for%20babies%20and%20young%20children

UKHSA 2023b Evaluation Framework tool and guidance TBA

United Nations (online): http://www.un.org/sustainabledevelopment/development-agenda/

WHO (2019) TIP Tailoring Immunization Programmes: http://apps.who.int/iris/bitstream/handle/10665/329448/9789289054492-eng.pdf

WHO (online) Vaccines and Immunization: http://www.who.int/health-topics/vaccines-and-immunization#tab=tab_1

Appendix 1 Resources

This section details resources for vaccinators and the public. Many resources and sources of information have been highlighted throughout the book.

World Health Organization (WHO)

- WHO Vaccines and immunization
- WHO global network of reliable vaccine information Vaccine Safety Net

The UK Schedule

The Green Book *Immunisation Against Infectious Diseases*

Provides information for public health professionals on immunisations, with sections on how vaccines work and principles of best practice and detail for each vaccine preventable disease
    Immunisation against infectious disease—GOV.UK

Vaccine Programme Guidance for Healthcare Practitioners
Available alongside the individual vaccine programmes
    Online via the UKHSA immunisation collection (Immunisation—GOV.UK)
    Country specific information

- Northern Ireland: The Health and Social Care Northern Ireland (HSCNI) public health directorate pages on vaccine preventable disease
- Scotland: Public Health Scotland Immunisation vaccine and preventable disease
- Wales: Public Health Wales Immunisation and Vaccines

Joint Committee in Vaccination (JCVI)
An expert scientific advisory committee with a statutory remit to advise the UK government on vaccination

Minutes for committee and subgroups: Joint Committee on Vaccination and Immunisation—GOV.UK

The Medicines and Healthcare Products Regulatory Agency
UK statutory agency responsible for the regulation of medicines, medical devices and blood components for transfusion in the UK
  Medicines and Healthcare products Regulatory Agency—GOV.UK

Electronic Medicines Compendium (EMC)
Provides up to date, approved and regulated prescribing and patient information for licensed medicines, the summary Product of characteristics (SmPC) and Patient Leaflet (PIL)
  https://www.medicines.org.uk/emc

Additional Resources—Grouped Under Themes

Vaccine Programmes and Vaccine Ingredients

- The UKHSA produces a range of leaflets on vaccination in general and the specific vaccine programmes—these are available to order free of charge and in a range of languages
  Via the Department of Health order line (Home—Health Publications)

Further information on vaccine ingredients and what is in vaccine

- National Health Service (NHS). Vaccinations
- National Health Service (NHS). Vaccinations and vaccine ingredients
- The Green Book Chapter 6: Contraindications and Special considerations
- UKHSA Use of human and animal products in vaccines—GOV.UK (www.gov.uk)
- The Oxford Vaccine Knowledge Vaccine ingredients | Vaccine Knowledge Project (ox.ac.uk)

Centers for Disease Control USA

- This page details how vaccines are developed and tested and undergo ongoing monitoring and surveillance (How Vaccines are Developed and Approved for Use | Vaccines & Immunizations | CDC).
- A table summarising vaccine excipients, by vaccine, used within the USA (many of which are also used within the UK) (https://www.cdc.gov/vaccines/pubs/pink-book/downloads/appendices/B/excipient-table-2.pdf).

To Support Assessing the Vaccines Needed by Those Under Vaccinated—To Catch Up
- Produced by UKHSA updated regularly (Vaccination of individuals with uncertain or incomplete immunisation)

Up to date information on specific country schedules. Vaccinators can use these to help compare and work out what the individual is missing.

- WHO immunisation data portal.
- European Centre for Disease Prevention and Control.
- US Centers for Disease Control (CDC) details vaccines and vaccine terms in other languages (foreign language translation tool).

Vaccines in Pregnancy
- UKHSA (2024) Pregnancy: how to help protect you and your baby
- Screening tests for you and your baby (STFYAYB)
- The Oxford Vaccine Knowledge Vaccination and Pregnancy | Vaccine Knowledge Project

Vaccines and Vaccine Preventable Diseases, Improving Uptake and Supporting Vaccine Conversations
- Oxford Vaccine Knowledge project—provides information and resources for vaccinators and to share with the public to help address queries. All information can be translated into many languages.
- JITSUVAX resources. Provide tools and information to help balance arguments and debunk vaccine disinformation.
- Vaccine Confidence Project, LSHTM: project monitoring confidence in vaccine programmes internationally—useful for current myths and controversies.
- National Institute for Health and Care Research NIHR Promoting vaccination: the right approach for the right group.
- British Society for Immunology https://www.immunology.org/.
- European Society for Disease Prevention and Control A collection of guides related to communicating about immunisation and communication toolkits on immunisation.

The following resources have information to support vaccine conversations but caution that these refer to US and Australian vaccine schedules.

- Children's Hospital of Philadelphia Vaccine Education Center
- Australian Academy of Science. The Science of Immunisation. Questions and Answers.
- Australian Sharing Knowledge About Immunisation (SKAI)

Traveller Health and Vaccines
- NATHNaC Travel Health Pro NaTHNaC—Factsheets (travelhealthpro.org.uk)
- Fitfortravel Home—Fit for Travel
- TRAVAX Home—TRAVAX (registration required)
- CDC Travellers' Health Yellow Book CDC Yellow Book 2024 | Travelers' Health | CDC

Appendix 2 Vaccinators: Best Practice/Scope of Practice Considerations

The word "vaccinators" is used here to describe anyone giving a vaccine. The following UKHSA documents provide further information on scope of practice UKHSA (2025) National Minimum Standards and Core Curriculum for Vaccination Training https://www.gov.uk/government/publications/national-minimum-standards-and-core-curriculum-for-immunisation-training-for-registered-healthcare-practitioners describes the standards for education and training for all vaccinators. The UKHSA (2025) Quality criteria for an effective Immunisation programme, https://www.gov.uk/government/publications/quality-criteria-for-an-effective-immunisation-programme provides guidance on the key elements required for the implementation and delivery of a safe, equitable, high quality, effective and efficient immunisation services.

Who Can Give a Vaccine? *Links to Chap. 4*

The Legalities: Safeguards and Governance Needed to Be in Place

- The law imposes a ***duty of care*** on anyone who delivers healthcare, at all levels and in any setting.
- The same standard of care would be expected of all practitioners performing a particular task or role.
- Employers and service managers are responsible for making sure their staff are appropriately trained and competent and that in the case of administering medicines, such as vaccines, they have the necessary legal authority in place.
- Practitioners are individually accountable for accepting any delegated work and responsible for their own actions.
- When delegating work to others or accepting work or delegating to others, individual practitioners need to consider the following:
  - **Ability**: Does the individual have the necessary skills and competence to do the work?

- **Accountability**: Is the work part of the individual's role/scope of practice/job description?
- **Authority**: Are appropriate local governance policies and protocols in place and the relevant legislation for medicine administration as detailed in the Human Medicines Regulations (HMR) (2012) adhered to, e.g. there can be no delegation under PGDs?

Development of Knowledge, Skills and Competence for Safe Vaccine Administration

All vaccinators should have completed core training and attend annual updates. The training content needs to include information on all the vaccines the vaccinator administers.

This training requirement is detailed in the following:

- National Minimum Standards and Core Curriculum for Immunisation Training for Registered Healthcare Practitioners. Details the core training for registered healthcare professional vaccinators involved in the delivery of all vaccines.
- Immunisation training of healthcare support workers: national minimum standards and core curriculum. Details the core training for non-registered healthcare support staff involved in adult vaccines, specifically influenza, pneumococcal and shingles vaccines.
- All vaccinators should complete a period of supervised practice and be assessed as having the necessary knowledge and skills and to be competent in vaccine administration.
- The RCN 2022 Immunisation knowledge and skills competence assessment tool provides a suitable framework to support this and also ongoing practice development.
- Vaccinators only administering influenza and/or COVID-19 vaccines—the training and assessment of competence in the Flu immunisation training recommendations and/or COVID-19: vaccinator training recommendations must be completed.

Medicine Administration *Links to Chap. 8*

The Human Medicines Regulations (HMR) (2012) governs the supply and administration of all medicines in the UK.

Prescription only medicines (POMs), which include all vaccines: supply and/or administration should ideally be undertaken on an individual patient specific basis with a prescription or a patient specific direction (PSD).

The HMR specify some exceptions which are available for certain situations and for some registered healthcare professionals, for example, patient group directions (PGDs) and national protocols.

Where a Vaccinator Cannot Use a PGD and a National Protocol Is Not an Option

- Vaccinators must only supply and/or administer vaccines in accordance with a patient specific direction (PSD).
- A PSD is often referred to as a prescription by those who write them, or use them, as the legal basis to administer a medication because this indicates that it is written by a prescriber.
- The PSD must be written and signed by an appropriate prescriber.
- The PSD can be an instruction from a prescriber to supply and/or administer a medicine to an individual patient or to a list of patients. The prescriber is responsible for the review and assessment for each individual patient

See Specialist Pharmacy Services Patient Specific Directions (PSD).

Is It Appropriate for the Vaccinator to Administer the Vaccine(s)?

The *prescriber* must be satisfied that the person to whom the administration is delegated has the qualifications, experience, knowledge and skills to provide the care or treatment involved.

The prescriber needs to consider the following:

- Is delegation in the best interest of the individual?
- Is the prescriber satisfied that the person to whom they delegate administration of the vaccine has the qualifications, experience, knowledge and skills needed?
- Has the vaccinator completed training in line with https://www.gov.uk/government/publications/nationalminimum-standards-and-core-curriculum-for-immunisation-training-for-registered-healthcare-practitioners to the National Minimum Standards and demonstrated been assessed as having the necessary knowledge, skills and competence?
- Is there adequate supervision and support in place on site?
- If working within their role and competence, is the vaccinator covered by their employer's vicarious liability or other employer or personal indemnity insurance?

If the answer to these questions is **NO**	If the answer to these questions is **YES**
It is **NOT** appropriate for the vaccinator to vaccinate. Consider further training, supervision and/or support mechanisms as appropriate.	The vaccinator **MAY** administer the vaccine, after considering: ✓ All health care professionals and support staff involved are accountable for their actions and practice. ✓ The prescriber needs to be satisfied that the vaccinator has the necessary skills and competence to administer the vaccine. ✓ The prescriber is accountable for the decision they made in delegating this task. ✓ The vaccinator is accountable for their practice during vaccine administration through civil law and to their employer.

MIX
Papier aus verantwortungsvollen Quellen
Paper from responsible sources
FSC® C105338

If you have any concerns about our products,
you can contact us on
ProductSafety@springernature.com

In case Publisher is established outside the EU,
the EU authorized representative is:
**Springer Nature Customer Service Center GmbH
Europaplatz 3, 69115 Heidelberg, Germany**

Printed by Libri Plureos GmbH
in Hamburg, Germany